Practical Management of Dementia

a multi-professional approach

Second Edition

Edited by

STEPHEN CURRAN

Consultant and Professor of Old Age Psychiatry
South West Yorkshire Partnership NHS Foundation Trust Wakefield
and School of Human and Health Sciences
University of Huddersfield

and

JOHN P WATTIS

Professor of Old Age Psychiatry
School of Human and Health Sciences
University of Huddersfield

Radcliffe Publishing
London • New York

Radcliffe Publishing Ltd
33–41 Dallington Street
London
EC1V 0BB
United Kingdom

www.radcliffepublishing.com

© 2011 Stephen Curran and John P Wattis

Stephen Curran and John P Wattis have asserted their right under the Copyright, Designs and Patents Act 1998 to be identified as the authors of this work.

All rights reserved. No part of this publication may be reproduced, stored in a retrieval system or transmitted, in any form or by any means, electronic, mechanical, photocopying, recording or otherwise, without the prior permission of the copyright owner.

British Library Cataloguing in Publication Data

A catalogue record for this book is available from the British Library.

ISBN-13: 978 184619 412 2

Typeset by Phoenix Photosetting, Chatham, Kent, UK
Cover designed by Tracey Thomas
Printed and bound by Cadmus Communications, USA

Contents

Preface to the second edition

Things change. Since the first edition of this book was published in 2004 we have seen a change of government in the UK and of president in the USA as well as a major collapse of financial markets. In the field of dementia management there have been changes, too. Social changes include an increasingly aged world population (Chapter 2) and rapidly changing government policies with increasingly meaningful engagement of patients and carers (Chapters 10, 15 and 16). The legal framework for managing issues of mental capacity in England and Wales has also been refined (Chapter 13).

Technological change has mostly been in the field of neuroimaging and other techniques to aid early diagnosis (Chapter 4), though some of these are presently too expensive or invasive for routine use. The usefulness and limitations of the cholinesterase inhibitors and memantine are better established and the *International Classification of Diseases* and the *Diagnostic and Statistical Manual of the American Psychiatric Association* are in a moderately advanced stage of revision, led in the case of dementia, by new research diagnostic criteria (Chapters 3 and 4). The neuropsychological underpinning of behavioural change in dementia is increasingly understood (Chapter 12).

Economic pressures are substantial and, in the UK at least, there seems to be increasing evidence that older people's mental health services are not receiving a fair share of the resources available for healthcare (Chapter 15).

Memory services are now well established. We have not tried to describe them here because of their variety and because the Memory Services National Accreditation Programme of the Royal College of Psychiatrists* has developed standards and an accreditation process that provides quality assurance for these diverse services.

So, although there has not been a major breakthrough in the pharmacological treatment of Alzheimer's disease or other forms of dementia, we thought it was time for a new edition of this work. We hope you agree!

Stephen Curran
John P Wattis
August 2011

---

* Royal College of Psychiatrists Memory Services National Accreditation Programme, www.rcpsych. ac.uk/quality/quality,accreditationaudit/memoryservices.aspx (accessed August 2011).

Preface to the first edition

In this book we have brought together findings from recent research with a multidisciplinary perspective into the practical aspects of dementia care. We strongly believe in the importance of bringing together the best in research and practice. When these are divorced, researchers may lose the vision of the real purpose of their work and practitioners may not have access to the most recent advances in knowledge. We hope this book will help bridge that gap. We have chosen our contributors mostly for their knowledge and practical experience in their own fields but also because of their expertise in policy and teaching. Looking after the needs of people with dementia demands a multi-talented, multidisciplinary approach. Practice in this field needs to be rooted in respect for the personhood of people with dementia. It needs to be underpinned by political support. Organisations like the Alzheimer's Society perform an invaluable function in campaigning on behalf of patients and their relatives. Nevertheless, issues like the closure of residential and nursing homes for largely financial reasons, despite the impact on residents, many of whom suffer from dementia, continue to cause concern.

If we ever develop dementia, we would like people to notice it early. We would like them to respect our autonomy but steer us quickly in the direction of the best help available. We would like to be seen by appropriately qualified people who could make a diagnosis and provide any useful medical treatment, social, psychological, nursing and therapy support and advice to ourselves and our families, and a truly personal approach to our needs, especially our spiritual needs. We hope this book will help people in developing the kind of services we would like to receive!

Stephen Curran
John P Wattis
January 2004

About the editors

Stephen Curran is Professor of Old Age Psychiatry, University of Huddersfield and Consultant in Old Age Psychiatry, South West Yorkshire Partnership NHS Foundation Trust, Wakefield. Stephen trained in Leeds and worked as Lecturer in Old Age Psychiatry at the University of Leeds until he took up his current post as Consultant in Old Age Psychiatry in Wakefield in 1998. His PhD research focused on Critical Flicker Fusion testing in people with dementia, a measure of information processing capacity. As well as running a busy old age psychiatry service he is also Lead Clinician for the Wakefield Memory Service and Chair of the Memory Services National Accreditation Programme Advisory Group at the Royal College of Psychiatrists.

John P Wattis is Professor of Old Age Psychiatry, University of Huddersfield. John was first appointed as a Consultant in Old Age Psychiatry in 1981. He held senior offices within the Faculty for Old Age Psychiatry of the Royal College of Psychiatrists and researched the development of the Specialty of Old Age Psychiatry. He has been R&D Director for several NHS Trusts. He is trained as a life coach and since his retirement from clinical work he has continued in his visiting university post, lecturing various student groups and supporting research. He has taught basic and advanced coaching skills to psychiatrists through the Royal College of Psychiatrists Education and Training Centre.

Contributors

Dorrie Ball, Senior Lecturer in Social Work, Huddersfield University, Queensgate, Huddersfield

Sue Barton, Deputy Director of Business Development, Fieldhead Hospital, Ouchthorpe Lane, Wakefield

Miguel A Bertoni, Consultant, East Kent Hospitals University NHS Foundation Trust; Senior Lecturer, University of Kent

Peter CW Bowie, Consultant and Clinical Director in Old Age Psychiatry, Sheffield Health and Social Care Trust, Fulwood House, Old Fulwood Road, Sheffield

Ben Boyd, General Manager, F Mill, Dean Clough, Halifax, West Yorkshire

Michael Carpenter, Consultant Physician for the Elderly, Pinderfields Hospital, Aberford Road, Wakefield

Richard Clibbens, Nurse Consultant, Older People's Services, Fieldhead Hospital, Ouchthorpe Lane, Wakefield

Stephen Curran, Consultant/Professor of Old Age Psychiatry, Fieldhead Hospital, Ouchthorpe Lane, Wakefield

Anthony Dearden, Consultant Old Age Psychiatrist, Leeds Partnership NHS Trust, Aire Court Community Unit, Lingwell Grove, Leeds

Arun Devasahayam, Specialist Registrar in Old Age Psychiatry, South West Yorkshire Partnership NHS Foundation Trust, Fieldhead Hospital, Wakefield

Mary Duggan, Senior Planning Manager, South West Yorkshire Partnership NHS Foundation Trust, Fieldhead Hospital, Wakefield

Nick Farrar, Service Co-ordination & Communications Manager, Bradford Metropolitan District Council, Olicana House, Chapel Street, Bradford

Abbie Flinders, Specialist Registrar in Medicine for the Elderly, Department of Medicine for the Elderly, St James's University Teaching Hospital, Leeds

Linda Harris, Chief Executive, Spectrum Community Health CIC, Union Street, Wakefield

Sonja Krüger, Specialist Registrar in Old Age Psychiatry, Leeds Partnership NHS Foundation Trust, Asket Croft, Asket Place, Leeds

Edgar Miller, Professor of Psychology, Department of Psychology, University of Leicester

Elizabeth Milwain, Freelance Psychologist Specialising in Later Life, Shipley, West Yorkshire

Virginia Minogue, Deputy Partnership Director, Joint Commissioning Unit, NHS Barnsley, Gateway Plaza, Barnsley

Shabir Musa, Consultant in Old Age Psychiatry, South West Yorkshire Partnership NHS Foundation Trust, Fieldhead Hospital, Wakefield

Anna V Richman, Consultant in Old Age Psychiatry, Mossley Hill Hospital, Merseycare NHS Trust, Liverpool

Jayanthi Devi Subramani, Specialist Registrar in Old Age Psychiatry, South West Yorkshire Partnership NHS Foundation Trust, Fieldhead Hospital, Wakefield

Daphne Wallace, Consultant in Old Age Psychiatry (retired), High Bentham, North Yorkshire via Lancaster

John P Wattis, Professor of Old Age Psychiatry, University of Huddersfield, School of Human and Health Sciences, Huddersfield

Ken CM Wilson, Professor of Old Age Psychiatry, Academic Unit, Elderly Mental Health Directorate, St Catherine's Hospital, Birkenhead

CHAPTER 1

Dementia in the new millennium

John P Wattis

A BRIEF HISTORY OF OUR UNDERSTANDING OF DEMENTIA

Dementia bears a stigma like other mental illnesses. Before effective pharmacological measures for mental illness were developed, that is before the last half of the last century, different models for understanding mental illness and different modes of treatment prevailed. The first positive post-medieval development was that of 'moral management' or 'moral treatment' of mental illness. Previously belief in demonology or views on the irrationality of people with mental illness had led to abuse and/or containment. Moral management brought about an engagement with the mentally ill person on an individual and collective level reflected in the modern Therapeutic Community movement. Reasoning and moral and emotional support produced good results in places like the Retreat in York, England and in other countries, too. The era of the large asylum and 'medicalisation' of mental illness followed. At the same time, the new discipline of psychoanalysis provided an explanation and treatment for some of the less severe mental disorders and had a wide impact on society. Critiques of an excessively medical model for understanding dementia[1] have led to practical measures of the well-being of patients with dementia[2] and recommendations for improved models of care.[3] Today, biological, social and psychological factors are all recognised as important in the management of dementia.

Although conditions described in Roman times probably correspond to current diagnoses of dementia, the modern *medical* history of the condition begins in 1906 when Alzheimer, a German neuropsychiatrist and associate of Kraeplin, described a woman in late middle age with the clinical picture and pathology of the disease that now bears his name. At another time, he also described the pathology of vascular dementia. At the time most cases of dementia in old people were written off as 'senile' dementia or 'senility'. Competing schools of neuropathology in Munich (Alzheimer) and Prague perpetuated this divide and the identity of Alzheimer's disease with most cases of 'senile' dementia was not widely realised for another half century.

In the mid-1950s Roth[4] published an account of the natural history of mental disorders in old age that distinguished between 'senile' and 'arteriosclerotic' psychosis on the basis of their outcomes. Further studies established the epidemiology of mental disorders in late life[5] and the quantitative pathology[6] of Alzheimer's and vascular dementia. The deficiency of the neurotransmitter acetylcholine in Alzheimer's disease was recognised 10 years later[7] and led to the development of the cholinergic hypothesis and therapies based on it. Initially these were based on attempts to increase the availability of choline by dietary supplementation with the precursor lecithin and subsequently on inhibition of the enzymes responsible for breaking down acetylcholine. In the meantime specialist mental health services for older people were developing and taking an interest in the positive management of people with dementia.[8] At this time Alzheimer's and vascular dementia were regarded as the two main causes of dementia, accounting singly or in combination for 90% or more of all cases (*see* Chapter 2). There were a host of other rarer causes such as Pick's disease and the 'metabolic' dementias of vitamin B_{12} and thyroid deficiency (*see* Chapter 6). More recently, diffuse Lewy body dementia has been recognised,[9] though it has still not been included in international diagnostic systems and there is still debate about its precise relationship with Alzheimer's disease, Parkinson's disease and other psychiatric disorders.[10,11] Often different types of pathology co-exist. The 'nun study' showed the importance of vascular damage in producing clinical dementia in patients with co-existing Alzheimer pathology,[12] confirming earlier pathological studies.

THE BURDEN OF DEMENTIA

Dementia imposes a terrible burden on society. The social burden is greatly influenced by demography since dementia is predominantly a condition of very old people. Since the beginning of the 20th century, the proportion of people in the United Kingdom (UK) over the age of 65 has risen threefold. The proportion of very old has increased even more markedly. Other countries in the developed world have been through similar changes and these changes are likely to be experienced in an accelerated way in the developing world (*see* Chapter 2).

Society may also increase the personal burden on people with dementia and those who care for them by the way it reacts to people with dementia (*see* Chapter 10) and by placing them and their carers under economic pressure. Political decisions about eligibility for care services supported by the state affect the financial burden. There is need for a debate about why old people with dementia should receive less favourable social support than young people with physical disability. For individuals afflicted with dementia the eventual loss of capacity for independent living threatens to take away their autonomy. For family and other carers there is the constant worry about safety and the burden of directly or indirectly meeting the needs of those who find it increasingly difficult to care for themselves. In the UK around three-quarters of a million people are currently affected.[13] In the United States (US) the comparable figure is around 5.3 million.[14] Currently between 18 and 37 million people worldwide are estimated to have one or other type of dementia and projections suggest that by 2025 this number will nearly double, with nearly three-quarters living in developing countries (*see* Chapter 2). The cost in terms of lost human potential and burden on caregivers is vast; current annual costs in the US alone are estimated at nearly $150 billion. Despite the fact that dementia is concentrated in late life it ranks 13th in the World Health Organization's list of causes of years lived with disability.[15] What can be done about so great a burden?

WHAT WE CAN DO?

We need to respond to the challenge at a variety of levels, including the following:
- ➤ the international level
- ➤ the national level
- ➤ the level of the local community
- ➤ the level of the family
- ➤ the personal level.

Internationally, organisations like Alzheimer's International, the World Health Organization and the International Psychogeriatric Association are trying to prepare countries in the developing world for the explosion in the prevalence of dementia that an ageing population will bring. In the developed world, there is still a need to eradicate ageist attitudes to the provision of support and treatment for people with dementia. At the population level, our developing knowledge of the risk factors for various forms of dementia may well enable us to produce a relative reduction in the numbers of people affected. For example, raised diastolic blood pressure has been linked to increased risk of memory impairment and cardiovascular health and brain health seem inextricably linked. Evidence is emerging that a Mediterranean diet, physical exercise and brain 'exercise' may all have a role in delaying the onset or progress of dementia. The inflammatory response to infection in older people with Alzheimer's disease may produce a permanent worsening of the cognitive state, possibly through inflammation-like reactions in the brain, suggesting that attention to the physical health of people with early dementia is especially important.

All these examples suggest immediate practical ways of reducing the population and individual risk of dementia. In addition, more fundamental genetic research is proceeding with three potentially important new genes reported in September 2009. These examples are taken from two months of reported research on the Alzheimer's Society website (www.alzheimers.org.uk and click through to 'research news').

However, *age* remains the greatest risk factor for developing dementia, especially Alzheimer's disease and so all those public health and lifestyle measures that increase longevity are likely to increase the population at risk. This does not mean we should give up. Reducing the prevalence of disease and its impact are fundamental tasks for medicine, related disciplines and the whole of society.

The 'ideal' scenario would be to develop the capacity to identify people at risk of dementia and to reduce that risk by acceptable and inexpensive public health or specific treatment measures. Genetic risk factors are already identified and will be discussed in more detail in Chapters 2 and 3. Measures to eliminate these genes from the gene pool are likely to be impractical, morally unacceptable and have unforeseeable consequences. However, genotyping to identify 'at risk' populations may, as our knowledge of the mechanisms of disease expands, enable preventive measures or early treatment at a pre-clinical stage before symptoms of disease develop. As new drugs are developed that interfere with the progression of Alzheimer's disease and as the population of the developing world ages dilemmas are likely to occur about the affordability of these drugs in poorer countries.

Local communities need to be helped to develop a better understanding of dementia and the issues that surround it so that families and people with dementia are treated as people and not marginalised. Old age psychiatry services, working through local government and primary care services, should see this education as one of their functions.

Families and individuals can take responsibility for lifestyle measures. At present avoiding smoking and excessive alcohol intake, a healthy diet, regular exercise, measures to reduce the risk of or treat high blood pressure and keeping the brain active can all be recommended as feasible ways of reducing risk. Once problems develop, positive management requires a bio-psycho-social model. A model that only considers one of these factors is wholly inadequate. Figure 1.1, taken from *Practical Psychiatry of Old Age*,[16] emphasises that in dealing with any individual patient we need to take into account brain, body, senses and physical and social environment *and the interaction between them*.

Positive management of dementia consists of first making a diagnosis and excluding rare, potentially treatable causes of dementia such as thyroid deficiency. Specific treatment for Alzheimer's dementia now exists and is probably effective in some other forms of dementia too, though use of the drugs in England is constrained by government guidelines.[17] The next step is to

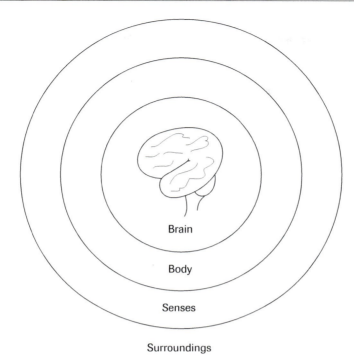

Brain

Body

Senses

Surroundings

Figure 1.1 An interactive model of confusion[16]

maximise the patient's capacity for independent living by optimising physical health, correcting deficiencies in hearing and sight and providing a supportive environment. Emotional and practical support to patients and carers requires collaboration across health and social care organisations. This kind of multi-layered approach fostered and was strengthened by the multidisciplinary approach to old age mental health services developed in the UK.[18-20] Other interventions, psychological and pharmacological, are required to cope with the depression and behavioural problems sometimes found in people with dementia.

However, even in the UK, one of the first countries to develop specific old age psychiatry services, there is a 'clinical iceberg'. The majority of people with dementia never come to the attention of those specialist services. There is a major need for specialist services to work together with primary care to improve access to those specialist services for people with dementia. The arrival of drugs for the treatment of Alzheimer's disease has increased the number of referrals and, in the UK, specialist memory clinics and services have increased in number to cope with increased demand.[21]

FUTURE DIRECTIONS

The first useful anti-dementia drugs, the cholinesterase inhibitors, have now been available for around 10 years. These drugs (donepezil, rivastigmine, galantamine and others) interfere with the breakdown of acetylcholine, effectively amplifying its effect at the synaptic cleft. Memantine, a drug with a completely different mode of action, has also been licensed in the UK for moderate to severe dementia of the Alzheimer type. Other existing drugs, such as the non-steroidal anti-inflammatory drugs, oestrogens and nicotine, may also have some effect on Alzheimer's dementia. It seems likely that anti-platelet drugs will help some patients with vascular dementia, though this has yet to be convincingly demonstrated. Drugs currently in development may affect the development of the insoluble form of beta amyloid by inhibiting some of the enzymes that split amyloid precursor protein. The immune system and inflammatory responses are important to our understanding of dementia, especially Alzheimer's disease. Other lines of enquiry, especially into the genetic risk factors for Alzheimer's and other dementias, are likely to suggest further therapeutic avenues. The herbal preparation, Gingko biloba, has also been shown to have some positive effect in Alzheimer's disease, though the mechanism of action is not clear. If we did understand it better, perhaps this too would suggest other lines of approach.

Nor does the future only lie in developing new drugs. Basic science may help us understand the processes that precede the clinical symptoms of Alzheimer's disease and may suggest preventative measures we cannot anticipate. Psychological and social care for people with dementia will develop. Indeed we could improve considerably on our current practical care for people with dementia by implementing what we already know and by educating those involved in providing care to people with dementia in the principles of person-centred care.[22] Improving the organisation and management of care should not be neglected either. This requires a more adequate political and social response to the challenges posed by an ageing society, including a more proportionate investment in dementia research and services for people with dementia. These were recognised in the UK by the National Dementia Strategy and parallel documents in Scotland, Wales and Northern Ireland[23] and new standards issued by the National Institute for Health and Clinical Excellence[24] (*see* Box 1.1). A new government in the UK, directly responsible for health services only in England, has endorsed the National Dementia Strategy, though it is hard to know yet whether the new vision of local accountability will work as well (or as poorly) as the old, more centralised model.

Box 1.1   NICE quality standards – indicators for quality dementia services

1   People with dementia receive care from staff appropriately trained in dementia care.

2   People with suspected dementia are referred to a memory assessment service specialising in the diagnosis and initial management of dementia.

3   People newly diagnosed with dementia and/or their carers receive written and verbal information about their condition, treatment and the support options in their local area.

4   People with dementia have an assessment and an ongoing personalised care plan, agreed across health and social care, that identifies a named care coordinator and addresses their individual needs.

5   People with dementia, while they have capacity, have the opportunity to discuss and make decisions, together with their carer(s), about the use of: advance statements, advance decisions to refuse treatment, lasting power of attorney, preferred priorities of care.

6   Carers of people with dementia are offered an assessment of emotional, psychological and social needs and, if accepted, receive tailored interventions identified by a care plan to address those needs.

7   People with dementia who develop non-cognitive symptoms that cause them significant distress, or who develop behaviour that challenges, are offered an assessment at an early opportunity to establish generating and aggravating factors. Interventions to improve such behaviour or distress should be recorded in their care plan.

8   People with suspected or known dementia using acute and general hospital inpatient services or emergency departments have access to a liaison service that specialises in the diagnosis and management of dementia and older people's mental health.

9   People in the later stages of dementia are assessed by primary care teams to identify and plan their palliative care needs.

10   Carers of people with dementia have access to a comprehensive range of respite/short-break services that meet the needs of both the carer and the person with dementia.

PRACTICAL MANAGEMENT OF DEMENTIA

The scope of what we currently can do is very wide and this book seeks to explore that scope. It does not look in detail at the anti-dementia drugs. We have asked contributors to cover epidemiology (the science of the distribution of disease in populations) and the current classification of the dementias into different diagnoses with different causes, time courses and (potentially) treatments. Building on that foundation, we have looked at the practical science of early detection and diagnosis. We have also taken a variety of perspectives: those of the psychiatrist, the clinical psychologist, the physician for the elderly, the general practitioner, the nurse, the occupational therapist and the social worker. We have explored the role of the 'memory clinic' and the special issues of early onset dementia. We have also asked contributors to discuss the legal framework in which we manage dementia (principally from the point of view of English law) and to share neglected but developing knowledge about the spiritual aspects of dementia and its management. Finally we have commissioned a chapter to discuss how comprehensive and integrated mental health services for people with dementia might be developed, rooted largely in practice in the UK. As in any edited work we are conscious of some repetitions, but in an effort to make each chapter reasonably self-sufficient we have not tried to eliminate these.

We are at the beginning of an exciting decade when major scientific advances in the diagnosis and management of Alzheimer's disease and other forms of dementia are likely to occur. These advances will require political commitment and financial support if they are to bear fruit in preventing or delaying the onset of dementia and in improving the quality of life of people with dementia and those who care for them. In the meantime, this book aims to be a useful practical guide to the current state of knowledge about the management of dementia. By approaching the problems of dementia from a multidisciplinary perspective we hope to stimulate the creativity of our readers in developing and implementing best practice in dementia care.

Key points

➤ The modern 'bio-medical' understanding of dementia is only a century old.

➤ It is inadequate without a broader 'psycho-social' approach.

➤ The burden on society from dementia is related to an ageing population.

➤ The burden on individuals with dementia and their carers is worsened by ageism manifested in reduced support when compared with chronic disabilities affecting younger people.

➤ International and national action is needed to meet the political and economic challenges of an ageing population and an increased prevalence of dementia.

➤ Local communities can respond with more understanding if old age services make education part of their task.

➤ Families and people with dementia can be helped by an integrated biological, psychological and social approach in a multidisciplinary framework.

➤ This book seeks to set out the current 'state of the art' of practical provision for people with dementia and aims to stimulate creative innovation.

REFERENCES

1 Kitwood T. The dialectics of dementia: with particular reference to Alzheimer's disease. *Ageing and Society.* 1990; **10**: 177–96.

2 Kitwood T, Bredin K. A new approach to the evaluation of dementia care. *Journal of Advances in Health and Nursing Care.* 1992; **1**(5): 41–60.

3 Kitwood T. *Dementia Reconsidered: the person comes first.* Buckingham: Open University Press; 1997.

4 Roth M. The natural history of mental disorder in old age. *Journal of Mental Science.* 1955; **101**: 281–301.

5 Kay DW, Beamish P, Roth M. Old age mental disorders in Newcastle-upon-Tyne; Part I: A study of prevalence. *British Journal of Psychiatry.* 1964; **110**: 146–58.

6 Blessed G, Tomlinson BE, Roth M. The association between quantitative measures of dementia and senile change in the grey matter of elderly people. *British Journal of Psychiatry.* 1968; **144**: 797–811.

7 Perry E, Tomlinson BE, Bergmann K, *et al.* Correlation of cholinergic abnormalities with senile plaques and mental test scores in senile dementia. *British Medical Journal.* 1978; **2**: 1457–9.

8 Arie T. The morale and planning of psychogeriatric services. *British Medical Journal.* 1971; **iii**: 166–70.

9 Forstl H, Burns A, Luthert P, *et al.* The Lewy-body variant of Alzheimer's disease: clinical and pathological findings. *British Journal of Psychiatry.* 1993; **162**: 385–92.

10 Byrne EJ. Diffuse Lewy body disease, spectrum disorder or variety of Alzheimer's disease? *International Journal of Geriatric Psychiatry.* 1992; **7**: 229–34.

11 Birkett P, Desouky A, Han L, *et al.* Lewy bodies in psychiatric patients. *International Journal of Geriatric Psychiatry.* 1992; **7**: 235–40.

12 Snowdon DA, Greiner LH, Mortimer JA, *et al.* Brain infarction and the clinical expression of Alzheimer disease. The Nun Study. *Journal of the American Medical Association.* 1997; **227**: 813–17.

13 Alzheimer's Society website. www.alzheimers.org.uk (accessed July 2011).

14 Alzheimer's Association. *Alzheimer's Disease Facts and Figures*. Available at: www.alz.org/ (accessed July 2011).

15 World Health Organization. *World Health Report*. Geneva: WHO; 2001.

16 Wattis J, Curran S. *The Practical Psychiatry of Old Age*. Oxford: Radcliffe Publishing; 2001.

17 National Institute for Clinical Excellence. *Donepezil, Galantamine, Rivastigmine and Memantine for the Treatment of Alzheimer's Disease (Review of NICE Technology Appraisal Guidance 111)*, NICE technology appraisal guidance 217. London: NICE; 2011.

18 Wattis JP, Wattis L, Arie TH. Psychogeriatrics: a national survey of a new branch of psychiatry. *British Medical Journal*. 1981; **282**: 1529–33.

19 Wattis JP. Geographical variations in the provision of psychiatric services for old people. *Age and Ageing*. 1988; **17**: 171–80.

20 Wattis J, Macdonald A, Newton P. Old age psychiatry: a specialty in transition – results of the 1996 survey. *Psychiatric Bulletin*. 1999; **23**: 331–5.

21 Lindesay J, Marudkar M, van Diepen E, *et al.* The second Leicester survey of memory clinics in the British Isles. *International Journal of Geriatric Psychiatry*. 2002; **17**: 41–7.

22 Kitwood T, Bredin K. *Person to Person: a guide to the care of those with failing mental powers*. Loughton: Gale Centre Publications; 1992.

23 Department of Health. *Living Well with Dementia: a national dementia strategy*. London: DoH; 2009.

24 National Institute for Health and Clinical Excellence. *Dementia Quality Standards*. London: NICE, 2010. www.nice.org.uk/aboutnice/qualitystandards/dementia/dementiaqualitystandard.jsp (accessed August 2011).

CHAPTER 2

Epidemiology of dementia

Peter CW Bowie

INTRODUCTION

Although dementia has been recognised for centuries it has only been the focus of scientific enquiry since Alois Alzheimer described the case of Auguste D just over 100 years ago. This chapter will discuss the demographic changes that have taken place since then, together with the prevalence and incidence of dementia and future changes in demography. The chapter will also discuss the current knowledge of risk factors for dementia and will emphasise the application of epidemiology and take a global as well as developed world view. However, first it is necessary to define dementia and its classification.

DEFINITIONS OF DEMENTIA

There have been various attempts to define dementia. For example, Roth[1] proposed that dementia is 'an acquired global impairment of intellect, memory and personality'. A more comprehensive definition has been suggested by McLean:[2] 'an acquired decline in a range of cognitive abilities (memory, learning, orientation and attention), and intellectual skills (abstraction, judgement, comprehension, language and calculation), accompanied by alterations in personality and behaviour which impair daily functioning, social skills and emotional control. There is no clouding of consciousness, and other psychiatric disorders are excluded.' The use of the term 'decline' is helpful because it emphasises the need for longitudinal assessment and a change from premorbid function. McKhann *et al.*[3] define dementia as 'the decline of memory and other cognitive functions in comparison with the patient's previous level of function as determined by a history of decline in performance and by abnormalities noted from clinical examination and neuro-psychological tests'. In addition, they suggest that diagnosis cannot be made when 'consciousness is impaired by delirium, drowsiness, stupor or coma, or when other clinical abnormalities prevent adequate evaluation of mental status'. More recently, definitions have been included in standardised diagnostic criteria including the *Diagnostic and Statistical Manual of the American Psychiatric Association, fourth edition (DSM-IV-TR)*[4] and the *International Classification of Diseases, 10th edition (ICD-10)*.[5] In the *ICD-10* definition, dementia is defined as:

> ... a syndrome due to disease of the brain, usually of a chronic or progressive nature, in which there is disturbance of multiple higher cortical functions, including memory, thinking, orientation, comprehension, calculation, learning capacity, language, and judgement. Consciousness is not clouded. Impairments of cognitive function are commonly accompanied, and occasionally preceded, by deterioration in emotional control, social behaviour or motivation.

Dementia can be classified in a number of different ways. For example, dementia can broadly be classified into reversible and irreversible forms. The irreversible dementias include early and late onset Alzheimer's disease, various forms of vascular dementia including multi-infarct dementia, Pick's disease, Creutzfeldt–Jakob disease, dementia with Lewy bodies, and dementia associated with Huntington's and Parkinson's disease and HIV.[5] These forms of dementia are progressive and usually lead to death. Traditionally, Alzheimer's disease has been thought to account for approximately 50% of all cases of dementia, with vascular dementia and mixed dementia (Alzheimer's disease and vascular dementia combined) each accounting for approximately 20% of all cases; the remaining 10% are due to reversible causes of dementia and less common primary brain degenerative diseases. The variation in the rates for underlying cause is often accounted for by the criteria used for diagnosis, for example, the NINDS-AIREN* criteria for vascular dementia are more stringent than the *ICD* or *DSM-IV* criteria and therefore a lower rate is reported when these criteria are used. It is also worth noting that there is a discrepancy between clinical diagnosis and pathological diagnosis.[6] In the last decade, there has been increasing interest in dementia with Lewy bodies, a condition characterised by fluctuating cognitive impairment, prominent hallucinations, Parkinsonism and falls. The condition is progressive and has pathological findings similar to Parkinson's disease.[7] It has been suggested that dementia with Lewy bodies is more common than vascular dementia, with prevalence studies reporting between 0 and 30.5% of dementia cases being due to dementia with Lewy bodies.[8] This wide variation in reported prevalence may be due to different diagnostic practices and a lack of distinction between dementia with

---

* National Institute of Neurological Disorders and Stroke and Association Internationale pour la Recherché et l'Enseignement en Neurosciences.

Lewy bodies and Parkinson's disease dementia. A review of the prevalence of Parkinson's disease dementia[9] suggests that 3.6% of dementia cases are due to Parkinson's disease dementia and that approximately 25% of Parkinson's disease cases are likely to have dementia.

A smaller number of patients have reversible dementia. The percentage of dementia patients with a reversible cause has varied from 8%[10] to 40%.[11] Byrne[12] defines 'reversible dementia' as 'the dementia syndrome that is caused by a potentially reversible or treatable condition'.

The potential reversibility of dementia is related to the underlying pathology and to the availability and application of effective treatment. The reversibility will be dependent on the initiating of treatment prior to irreversible damage occurring. Equally, some causes may be arrestable rather than reversible.

THE AGEING POPULATION

Since dementia is primarily a disease of the elderly, a clear understanding of the demographics of ageing can be used to facilitate projections of the epidemiology of dementia and allow for planning of service to meet future needs. The growth of elderly populations poses challenges to services, which must adapt provision to provide for the changing age structures of society.

The global population aged 65 and over was estimated to be 420 million in the year 2000, representing an increase of 9.5 million since 1999.[13] In 1990, 26 nations had elderly populations of more than 2 million and by 2000, 31 countries had reached the 2 million figure. Projections to the year 2030 indicate that more than 60 nations will have in excess of 2 million people aged 65 or over.[13] Table 2.1 shows estimates of the percentage of the population aged 65 and over by world region and projections from 2000 to 2030.

Percentages alone do not express a sense of the momentum of population growth. For example, while the increase in elderly populations in Sub-Saharan Africa from 2000 to 2015 is only 0.3%, this actually represents an increase of 9.6 million from an elderly population 19.3 to 28.9 million.

From 1970 to 1996 the percentage of the elderly population of Japan grew from 7% to 14%. Similar rapid increases are expected in South Korea, Taiwan, Thailand and China, fuelled by dramatic drops in fertility levels. This speed of change can be contrasted with Europe and North America where comparable increases took place over 100 years.

Increases in life expectancy partly account for the changing demographics of the elderly. This, in conjunction with lowering birth rates, results in a higher proportion of the population being aged 65 and over. Expansion of public healthcare and disease eradication programmes greatly increased life expectancy in the second half of the 20th century, and from 1900 to 1950 people in the developed world were able to add 20 years or more to their life expec-

Table 2.1 Percentage of the population aged 65 and over by world region

Region	Year	65 years +
Europe	2000	15.5
	2015	18.7
	2030	24.3
North America	2000	12.6
	2015	14.9
	2030	20.3
Oceania	2000	10.2
	2015	12.4
	2030	16.3
Asia	2000	6.0
	2015	7.8
	2030	12.0
Latin America/Caribbean	2000	5.5
	2015	7.5
	2030	11.6
Near East/North Africa	2000	4.3
	2015	5.3
	2030	8.1
Sub-Saharan Africa	2000	2.9
	2015	3.2
	2030	3.7

tancy.[13] Throughout the world there are variations in life expectancy, with people in Japan and Singapore being currently expected to live the longest, around 80 years, whilst many African countries stand at only 45 years.[13] Life expectancy for someone born today in the developed world is, on average, 70.9 years, with the UK standing at 77.7 years and the US at 77.1 years. The average life expectancy for someone born in the developing world is harder to summarise, with estimates ranging from 80.1 years in Singapore (currently the highest) to 37.6 years in Malawi and Zimbabwe.

In general, women outlive men. The UK Census 2001 revealed that the life expectancy of a female born in the UK in 2001 was 80 years, with males expecting to live 75 years.[14] Similar age-related differences were found worldwide.[13]

In summary, the world's population aged 65 and over is growing by approximately 800 000 people per month.[13] Global ageing is occurring at a pace never seen before, and this rapid increase will be reflected in the epidemiology of age-related diseases such as dementia. One prediction for Alzheimer's disease in the US is that the population affected will quadruple in the next 50 years.[15] Predictions for the period 2001 to 2040 suggest that whilst developed nations will see nearly a 200% increase in prevalence, many developing nations will experience an increase of over 300%, with Latin America and North Africa seeing increases in prevalence close to 400%.[16]

PREVALENCE AND INCIDENCE OF DEMENTIA

Prevalence refers to the number of people with dementia at the given point in time.[17] Prevalence rates vary enormously and some of the reasons for this have been reviewed by Henderson and Kay.[18] As the sample size increases, prevalence estimates become more accurate. Prevalence is also influenced by the sample composition. For example, community samples generally give lower prevalence rates compared with residential homes since the latter tend to cater specifically for patients with dementia. The number of elderly and very elderly in the denominator is also an important factor.

As the number of elderly people in the general population increases, so does the prevalence of dementia, with rates rising from 2.1% between 65 and 69 years to 17.7% in those aged 80 years or above. Thus, prevalence rates will vary depending on the geographical location of the study. For similar reasons, they will also be influenced by when the study was conducted because the number of elderly in the general population has been gradually increasing over the last 100 years. Diagnostic criteria are also very important in that the more rigid the diagnostic criteria become, the smaller the prevalence of the condition. Finally, the type of prevalence study has a major effect on the prevalence rate. Period prevalence (the number of cases in a given population during a specified period), compared with point prevalence studies (the number of cases in a given population at a specific time), will produce higher prevalence rates since period prevalence is technically a combination of prevalence and incidence.

Incidence is the number of new cases occurring in a given population during a specified time period,[17] and is generally regarded as a more useful indicator than prevalence. This is partly because differences in prevalence rates could be due to either differences in the number of new cases or differences in survival rates. Despite this, there have been considerably fewer studies of incidence. Incidence rate is relatively small and 'in order to yield reliable data' studies either need to be very large or conducted over many years. A review and meta-analysis of studies[19] showed that incidence rates increase with increasing age but the incidence rate ratio (the rate of change of the incidence) slows down with increasing age, for example, the incidence rate triples from 60 to 65 years, but increases by only a factor of 1.5 from 80 to 85 years. The incidence rate ratio does not fall below one so there is no evidence that the rate eventually begins to decline. The incidence rates for five-year age groups are shown in Table 2.2. The reason for the levelling off of the incidence of dementia in the very old is unknown.

Table 2.2 Annual incidence of dementia from 12 studies[19]

Age group	Annual incidence rate (%)
55–59	0.033
60–64	0.11
65–69	0.33
70–74	0.84
75–79	1.82
80–84	3.36
85–89	5.33
90–94	7.23

Gender did not appear to be a significant factor in the incidence of dementia; women are at higher risk for developing an incidence of Alzheimer's disease whilst men are at higher risk for vascular dementia.[19] Gender does not appear to be a factor in the incidence of dementia with Lewy bodies, but studies have been too small to draw absolute conclusions.[8]

Prevalence by age

The exact prevalence of dementia is unknown and is influenced by a number of different factors. Kay and Bergman[20] reported that the prevalence of dementia gradually increases with increasing age: 2.1% are affected between the ages of 65 and 69 and this rises to 17.7% in those aged 80 or above. Jorm and Jolley[21] suggest, following a meta-analysis of 23 studies, that the prevalence rises exponentially with age, doubling with each successive period of 5.1 years. These findings were confirmed in later studies.[22–24] A summary of the prevalence rates is shown in Table 2.3. There are some inconsistencies concerning prevalence of dementia in extreme old age (aged 90 onwards). Jorm[25] suggested that the risk of developing dementia declines in extreme old age. However, later, Jorm and Jolley[21] found no decrease in extreme old age, suggesting that everybody will develop dementia if they live long enough.

Table 2.3 Age-specific prevalence of dementia averaged from 18 studies[21]

Age group	Prevalence rate %
65–69	1.4
70–74	2.8
75–79	5.6
80–84	10.5
85–89	20.8
90–95	38.6

Prevalence by gender

There is invariably a preponderance of females in any demented population, though this largely reflects the greater number of elderly females in the general population. Indeed, the excess of females in 'post-mortem confirmed Alzheimer's disease' is consistent with the age-matched male to female ratio in the general population.[26] Overall, there were no age-specific sex differences in prevalence rates for dementia. However, the prevalence rate of Alzheimer's disease is generally higher amongst females when compared with males of the same age.[27]

Prevalence by geographical area

The reported prevalence and incidence of dementia varies enormously throughout the world. These differences may, in part, be explained by methodological differences, including different diagnostic criteria, screening methods and statistical analyses. However, these differences may also be explained by true differences in the incidence of dementia, the progress of the disease and differential survival rates. Although a great deal of work has been done throughout the world, research conducted in the UK and Ireland; the US and developing countries including Asia, the Far East, Latin America, and Africa will be discussed in more detail in the following sections.

United Kingdom and Ireland

The first major study of the prevalence of dementia in the UK was undertaken by Sheldon[28] in Wolverhampton following World War II. More recent studies have been undertaken in Newcastle,[29] London[30] and Dublin.[31] The prevalence rates obtained vary significantly from 2.3% of over 65-year-olds to 17.5% of over 80-year-olds. It appears, however, that this variation in prevalence is partly due to differences in the prevalence of different types of dementia, with the onset age for vascular dementia being lower than that of Alzheimer's disease.[32] An overall rate of 5% is suggested.[33]

The United States

Similar rates to those obtained in the UK have been seen in North America,[34] with approximately 5% of those aged over 65 suffering from dementia.

In the US, an interesting area of research is ethnic differences. The majority of studies in the US have, however, focused on predominantly white populations. An exception to this is a study by Perkins *et al.*[35] who screened white, Hispanic and black retired men in Houston. They found a difference in the prevalence of dementia relating to ethnic group. Hispanic and black men were found to be at highest risk, with prevalence of 4.75% and 4.80% respectively, whilst white men had a prevalence of 2.42%. However, it should be noted that a higher incidence of strokes, hypertension and diabetes are found in African-Americans and this could partly account for the higher prevalence of dementia, especially given that the Perkins *et al.*[35] study found 55% of their participants being diagnosed with vascular dementia, with only 20% having Alzheimer's disease. More detailed work is required, therefore, to fully understand the link between ethnicity and geographical area with respect to dementia.

Developing countries: Asia and the Far East

An interesting pattern has been obtained in the Far East. In the past, Chinese culture has associated the appearance of dementia with retribution for past sins, the imbalance of Yin and Yang and a consequence of astrological activity.[36] Such beliefs may result in dementia being seen not as an illness, and the help of Chinese healers rather than Westernised medical help being sought. Rapid urbanisation is, however, being shown to be resulting in changing family structure in the Far East, such as smaller family sizes in China, and the beliefs regarding dementia have also been shown to be becoming more 'westernised'.[36]

There have been a number of studies looking at prevalence rates in older people with dementia. Many early studies in the Far East yielded low prevalence rates.[37] Later studies, however, adopting a rigorous methodology, indicated a prevalence rate of around 5%.[38,39] More recent studies using validated case finding tools devised for use in developing countries have suggested that conventional diagnostic criteria may lead to an underestimation of the prevalence of dementia.[40] These studies, using the 10/66 dementia algorithm,[41] suggested prevalence rates of 6.3% in urban China and 3.5% in rural China compared with rates of 3.1% and 2% respectively according to *DSM-IV* criteria. Similar diagnostic discrepancies were also found in India, where according to the 10/66 criteria prevalence was 2.1% in urban areas and 1.4% in rural areas compared with 0.9% and 0.3% respectively using *DSM-IV* criteria. Alzheimer's disease appears to be the predominant cause of dementia in China, accounting for approximately two-thirds of cases.[42]

Japan, a country with one of the highest life expectancies, had one million dementia sufferers in 1990, and the number of sufferers was estimated to double by 2010.[43] The incidence of vascular dementia in Japan[44] was greater than the incidence of Alzheimer's disease, with double the rate for men and similar rates for women. More recently Yamada *et al.*[45] have found that this picture has reversed and Alzheimer's disease is twice as prevalent as vascular dementia. In addition they also found a significant number of cases of dementia with Lewy bodies, but these did not match the rates for vascular dementia (2.8% and 28% of cases respectively).

Developing countries: Latin America

The prevalence of dementia in Latin American countries has only recently been studied.[40] Again, marked discrepancies were found in prevalence rates depending on diagnostic criteria. Using the 10/66 diagnostic algorithm, prevalence rates varied from 7.3% in urban areas to 3.8% in rural areas. Using *DSM-IV* criteria, prevalence estimates were 4.4% and 1.8% respectively.

Developing countries: Africa

The majority of the work on dementia in Africa has been conducted in Nigeria. Research has included community surveys, hospital admission studies and autopsy studies. Three separate community surveys, with approximately 23 000 participants, have found no cases of dementia.[46–48] It has been suggested that the nil rate may be due to a number of different factors, particularly the lower life expectancy, and also African families being tolerant of disturbed behaviour, a reluctance to seek psychiatrists' help, a preference for the use of African medicine and a fear of stigmatisation. American psychiatrists conducted a study that found a prevalence rate of 2.29% for dementia and 1.41% for Alzheimer's alone.[49] Interestingly, however, this study was extended to include a comparison group of Nigerians living in the US. Significantly higher prevalence rates for dementia and Alzheimer's disease were obtained for the US population of 8.24% and 6.24%.[50] This finding suggests the involvement of environmental factors in the aetiology of dementia.

Temporal changes in the prevalence of dementia

Two major studies have investigated the prevalence of dementia over time. The Lundby study in Sweden followed prevalence of dementia from 1947 to 1972, and showed no change in prevalence of either multi-infarct or what was described as 'senile dementia'.[51] Similarly, no change in prevalence was obtained in Rochester, US from 1975 to 1980.[52] However, Kokmen *et al.*[53] found an increase in the cases of dementia in Rochester between 1960 and 1984.

Suh and Shah[54] conducted a meta-analysis of all publications on the epidemiology of dementia from 1966 to 1999. Overall they concluded that the prevalence of dementia had increased and it appeared that when dementia was separated into Alzheimer's disease and vascular dementia for the purposes of analysis, temporal changes could be seen. The prevalence of the two types was found to vary throughout the world. Although these differences may be partly due to methodological differences, they may, however, reflect true differences in the incidence, differential survival and mortality after the onset of dementia. A difference in the prevalence of dementia in Korea, China and Japan was observed, with vascular dementia being more common in the 1980s whilst Alzheimer's disease was more common in the 1990s.

RISK FACTORS FOR DEMENTIA

As we have already discussed, the prevalence of dementia and especially Alzheimer's disease increases exponentially with increasing age, thus age is by far the biggest risk factor for dementia. Relatively few risk factors have been conclusively established, although many have been considered. Most of the evidence on risk factors has been based on case-control studies, but large longitudinal cohort studies have now been published which avoid some of the methodological problems associated with case-control studies.

Family history of Alzheimer's disease and other dementias has been associated with a risk for Alzheimer's disease in most studies, but not all. A number of genes have been identified as being associated with Alzheimer's disease – mutations of genes on chromosomes 1, 14 and 21 are linked with early-onset familial Alzheimer's disease, but together these genes account for fewer than 2% of all cases. The vast majority of cases are late-onset and so far the only confirmed genetic marker associated with late-onset risk is the ε4 allele of apolipoprotein E (APOE), a protein encoded on chromosome 19.[55] There are three allelic variants of APOE ε: ε2, ε3 and ε4; ε3 is the most frequent allele found in the general population, with frequency estimates ranging from 63% to 85%; ε2 is comparatively rare (3%–13%) and ε4 frequencies range from 7% to 29%. People who are ε4 homozygotes (possess two ε4 alleles) are at particular risk of developing Alzheimer's disease, with 50% to 90% of such individuals eventually developing the disease. Those with one ε4 allele also carry an increased risk, with 29% eventually developing the disease. Those individuals without the ε4 allele have a lifetime risk of about 9%.[56] Homozygosity for APOE ε4 has also been linked to a faster rate of cognitive decline, suggesting that the protein has a mechanistic role in disease progression and is not simply related to disease onset.[57] Other genes have been linked to sporadic Alzheimer's, with findings relating to chromosome 12 being the most compelling. However, so far the evidence for this remains inconclusive.

There is substantial evidence that a history of head injury increases the risk of Alzheimer's disease, although some studies have not found an association.[58,59] It has been well established that head injury is associated with a massive increase in amyloid in the brain, and it is the brain's ability to deal with this increased amyloid burden that is the likely mechanism for any increased risk.

Other factors associated with increased risk for Alzheimer's disease are less well established. Family history of brain disease and parental age have both been studied; both reflect possible exposure to genetic factors. Family history of Parkinson's disease and Down's syndrome have been studied with inconsistent results.[60,61] Likewise, maternal age at birth has not consistently been associated with an increased risk of dementia. Other medical conditions such as allergic conditions, hypothyroidism and viral infection do not have a consistent association with Alzheimer's disease.[62]

Environmental and lifestyle factors have also been studied. Aluminium has been researched for many years, but there is still not conclusive evidence that it has a causal role in Alzheimer's disease.[63] Smoking has been widely studied: earlier case-control studies suggested that smoking may reduce the risk for Alzheimer's disease but more recent longitudinal cohort studies have shown no effect or an increased risk.[64] A study looking at the combined effect of smoking, drinking and exercise suggested that these factors were not associated with risk for Alzheimer's disease.[65] Results from a Canadian cohort study involving over 6000 subjects suggested that regular physical activity and use of wine, coffee and non-steroidal inflammatory drugs were associated with a reduced risk of Alzheimer's disease;[66] the authors suggested that these factors required further investigation.

Other lifestyle factors to be considered include diet and obesity. The low risk of developing dementia in developing countries may be attributable to diet. Diets rich in fruit, vegetables and fibre may reduce neuropathological processes and may contribute to the low prevalence findings in Nigeria and in parts of Asia.[42] Other dietary factors may increase risk, for example, tofu consumption has been associated with cognitive decline in Japanese Americans;[67] and consumption of the cycad fruit is associated with the development of the Parkinson dementia complex prevalent in Guam.[68] Obesity in middle age was highlighted as a risk factor in the 27-year follow-up of a large North American cohort. Obesity (body mass index > 30) was found to increase risk by 74%, whilst being overweight (body mass index 25–29.9) increased risk by 35% compared with those with normal weight (body mass index 18.6–24.9).[69]

Vascular risk factors such as hypertension, hypercholesterolaemia and atherosclerosis have been shown to increase the risk for Alzheimer's disease and dementia generally.[70]

Other factors have been associated with a reduced risk for developing Alzheimer's disease. The most consistent evidence is regarding higher educational attainment and length of education, which are associated with a lower risk.[71] Stern and colleagues[72] postulated two mechanisms of cognitive reserve that might explain the finding. The first hypothesis suggests that pre-existing brain networks may be more resilient and less susceptible to disruption. The second hypothesis suggests alternative neural networks may compensate for the disruption caused by pathological change.

The use of various medications and vitamins has been explored. Anti-inflammatory drugs, statins, hormone replacement therapy (HRT) and vitamins C and E have all been studied as potential agents that could reduce the risk of developing dementia in late life. In a prospective cohort study of nearly 7000 subjects followed up for seven years, Veld et al.[73] found that short-term use of non-steroidal anti-inflammatory drugs was associated with a relative risk of Alzheimer's disease of 0.95, whilst long-term use was associated with a relative risk ratio of 0.2. Use of non-steroidal anti-inflammatory drugs did not reduce the risk of vascular dementia. In a nested case-control study, Jick et al.[74]

found that the adjusted relative risk (odds ratio) of developing dementia was 0.29 for those prescribed statins. This finding was independent of the presence or absence of untreated hyperlipidaemia. However, a more recent systematic review of large controlled trials of statins did not show any beneficial effect in terms of preventing future cognitive decline[75] and, despite the biological feasibility that statins might be protective, the current evidence suggests statins have no effect in preventing dementia. Early studies of HRT suggested that HRT mitigates the degeneration that leads to Alzheimer's disease. However, a large-scale randomised trial, the Women's Health Initiative Memory Study,[76] found that participants taking HRT were more at risk of cognitive decline and dementia than those taking a placebo. Current evidence, therefore, does not support the use of HRT to reduce the risk of future dementia. Two large longitudinal cohort studies suggested that antioxidant use (vitamins C and E) was associated with a reduced risk of Alzheimer's disease. Engelhart et al.[77] followed up over 5000 participants for six years and found, after adjusting for confounders, a significantly reduced risk in those using vitamin C and vitamin E – this finding was independent of APOE ε status. The other study[78] followed a cohort of 815 participants for nearly four years and found that increased vitamin E intake was associated with a lower risk for Alzheimer's disease; however, this finding was only observed in those people who were APOE ε4 negative.

Lastly, there is the question of depression, which is associated with cognitive impairment in older people.[79] Case-control studies have suggested an association between a history of depression and risk for Alzheimer's disease.[80] However, longitudinal studies have been inconsistent.[81,82]

DISCUSSION

A major problem in epidemiological studies of dementia is defining a case. This is especially true for mild cases of dementia, particularly when combined with poor education or lower IQ.[83] In addition, there are difficulties when using informants,[84] which may be particularly true in developing countries. Informants may have a tendency to offer responses perceived to be acceptable to the interviewer, may expect questions to be addressed to the head of the family/tribe, and personal questions may be avoided. In developing countries, reporting of age has been shown to be inaccurate, with the under-reporting by three years being observed in elderly Indian patients,[85] while Chinese informants tend to add an extra year.[86]

Some techniques of case identification are less reliable than others. For example, hospital admission is not a reliable index of dementia cases as the majority of patients are likely to be nursed at home, particularly in developing countries. Geographical comparison based on hospital admission is a reflection of service provision rather than prevalence of dementia.[87]

Despite such methodological concerns, the study of the epidemiology of dementia is crucial. As the age distribution of the world population shifts, dementia is emerging as a major health problem. The assessment of epidemiology of the disease provides crucial input for public health professionals in determining and allocating healthcare resources. The increasing burden of care for families has to be taken on by governmental response. Issues to be addressed by governments include the extent of domiciliary, day and residential care that should be available in order to provide the appropriate level of support for both sufferers and their families. Owing to the increasing life expectancy, the number of people suffering from dementia will rise steeply over the next decades. Additional importance must be given to planning for the care of the elderly and to account for the likely dramatic increase of dementia sufferers in the future. In addition, strategies to reduce risk must be sought, evaluated and implemented. Dementia can be seen as a problem today and a likely epidemic tomorrow.

Key points

➤ The work reviewed in this chapter provides an overview of the prevalence and incidence of dementia across the world, and considers possible risk factors associated with disease onset.

➤ Epidemiology has enormous potential for identifying modifiable risk factors and ways to prevent disease.

➤ Further advances in the understanding of dementia are required, and epidemiological studies have been of use in providing such insights.

➤ Further intensive studies into areas where rates appear very high or low may prove fruitful in furthering research into the aetiology of dementia.

REFERENCES

1 Roth M. The natural history of mental disorder in old age. *Journal of Mental Science.* 1955; **101**: 281–301.

2 McLean S. Assessing dementia. Part 1: Difficulties, definitions and differential diagnosis. *Australian & New Zealand Journal of Psychiatry.* 1987; **21**: 142–74.

3 McKhann G, Drachman D, Folstein M, *et al.* Clinical diagnosis of Alzheimer's disease: Report of NINCDS-ADRDA Work Group under the auspices of Department of Health and Human Services Task Force on Alzheimer's disease. *Neurology.* 1984; **34**: 939–44.

4   American Psychiatric Association. *Diagnostic and Statistical Manual of Mental Disorders.* 4th ed. Washington, DC: APA; 2000.

5   World Health Organization. *The ICD-10 Classification of Mental and Behavioural Disorders.* Geneva: WHO; 1992.

6   Knopman DS, DeKosky ST, Cummings JL, *et al.* Practice parameter: diagnosis of dementia (an evidence-based review). Report of the Quality Standards Subcommittee of the American Academy of Neurology. *Neurology.* 2001; **56**: 1143–53.

7   McKeith IG, Galasko D, Kosaka K, *et al.* Consensus guidelines for the clinical and pathologic diagnosis of dementia with Lewy bodies (DLB): report of the consortium on DLB international workshop. *Neurology.* 1996; **47**: 1113–24.

8   Zaccai J, McCracken C, Brayne C. A systematic review of prevalence and incidence of dementia with Lewy bodies. *Age and Ageing.* 2005; **34**: 561–66.

9   Aarsland D, Zaccai J, Brayne C. A systematic review of prevalence studies of dementia in Parkinson's disease. *Movement Disorders.* 2005; **20**: 1255–63.

10 Pearce J, Miller E. *Clinical Aspects of Dementia.* London: Baillere Tindall; 1973.

11 Hutton JT. Senility reconsidered. *Journal of the American Medical Association.* 1981; **245**: 1025–6.

12 Byrne EJ. Diffuse Lewy-body disease: disease spectrum disorder or variety of Alzheimer's disease. *International Journal of Geriatric Psychiatry,* 1987; **7**: 229–34.

13 Kinsella K, Velkoff V. *An Ageing World: 2001.* International population reports: US Department of Health and Human Sciences, National Institute of Health. Washington DC: United States Census Bureau; 2001.

14 Office for National Statistics. *Social Trends.* London: HMSO Publications; 2001.

15 Brookmeyer R, Gray S, Kawas C. Projections of Alzheimer's disease in the United States and the public health impact of delaying disease onset. *American Journal of Public Health.* 1998; **88**: 1337–42.

16 Ferri CP, Prince M, Brayne C, *et al.* Global prevalence of dementia: a Delphi consensus study. *Lancet.* 2005; **366**: 2112–17.

17 Barker DJP, Rose G. *Epidemiology in Medical Practice,* 4th ed. London: Churchill Livingstone; 1990.

18 Henderson AS, Kay DWK. The epidemiology of mental disorders in the aged. In: Kay DWK, Burrows GD (eds). *Handbook of Studies on Psychiatry and Old Age.* Amsterdam: Elsevier; 1984.

19 Gao S, Hendrie HC, Hall KS, *et al.* The relationships between age, sex, and the incidence of dementia and Alzheimer disease: a meta-analysis. *Archives of General Psychiatry.* 1998; **55**: 809–15.

20 Kay DWK and Bergman K. Epidemiology of mental disorders among the aged in the community. In: Birren JE, Sloane RB (eds). *Handbook of Mental Health and Ageing,* Englewood Cliffs, NJ: Prentice-Hall; 1980.

21 Jorm AF, Jolley D. The incidence of dementia: a meta-analysis. *Neurology.* 1998; **51**(3): 728–33.

22 Rocca WA, Hofman A, Brayne C, *et al.* Frequency and distribution of Alzheimer's disease in Europe: a collaborative study of 1980–1990 prevalence findings. The EURODEM-Prevalence Research Group. *Annals of Neurology.* 1991; **30**: 381–390.

23 Copeland JRM, Davidson IA, Dewey ME, *et al.* Alzheimer's disease, other dementias, depression and pseudo-dementia: prevalence, incidence and three year outcome in Liverpool. *British Journal of Psychiatry.* 1992; **161**: 230–9.

24 von Strauss E, Viitanen M, De Ronchi D, *et al.* Aging and the occurrence of dementia: findings from a population-based cohort with a large sample of nonagenarians. *Archives of Neurology.* 1999; **56**: 587–92.

25 Jorm AF. Cross-national comparisons of the occurrence of Alzheimer's and vascular dementias. *European Archives of Psychiatry and Clinical Neuroscience.* 1991; **240**: 218–22.

26 Heston LL, Mastri AR, Anderson VW, *et al.* Dementia of the Alzheimer type. Clinical genetics, natural history and associated conditions. *Archives of General Psychiatry.* 1981; **38**: 1085–90.

27 Jorm AF, Korten AE, Henderson AS. The prevalence of dementia; a quantitative integration of the literature. *Acta Psychiatrica Scandinavica.* 1987; **76**: 465–79.

28 Sheldon JH. *The Social Medicine of Old Age.* London: Oxford University Press; 1948.

29 Newens AJ, Forster DP, Kay DW, *et al.* Clinically diagnosed presenile dementia of the Alzheimer type in the Northern health region: ascertainment, prevalence, incidence and survival. *Psychological Medicine.* 1993; **23**: 631–44.

30 Livingstone G, Hawkins A, Graham N. The Gospel Oak study: prevalence rates of dementia and depression and activity limitation among elderly residents in Inner London. *Psychological Medicine.* 1990; **20**: 137–46.

31 Lawler BA, Radic A, Bruce I. Prevalence of mental illness in an elderly community dwelling population using AGECAT. *Irish Journal of Psychological Medicine.* 1994; **11**: 157–9.

32 Brayne C, Calloway P. An epidemiological study of dementia in a rural population of elderly women. *British Journal of Psychiatry.* 1989; **155**: 214–19.

33 Ineichen B. The geography of dementia: an approach through epidemiology. *Health and Place.* 1998; 4(4): 383–94.

34 Henderson AS. *Dementia.* Geneva: World Health Organization; 1994.

35 Perkins P, Annegars JF, Doody RS, *et al.* Incidence and prevalence of dementia in a multiethnic cohort of municipal retirees. *Neurology.* 1997; 49(1): 44–50.

36 Elliott KS, Di Minno M, Lam D. Working with Chinese families in the context of dementia. In: Yeo G, Gallagher-Thompson D (eds). *Ethnicity and the Dementias.* Washington, DC: Taylor and Francis; 1996. pp. 89–108.

37 Kua EH. The prevalence of dementia in elderly Chinese. *Acta Psychiatrica Scandinavica.* 1991; **83**: 350–2.

38 Chiu HFK, Pang AHT, Lam LCW, *et al.* Letter from Hong Kong. *International Journal of Geriatric Psychiatry.* 1996; **11**: 711–13.

39 Yang C-H, Hwang J-P, Tsai S-J. Types and phenomenologic subtypes of dementia in Taiwan: a psychiatric inpatient study. *International Journal of Geriatric Psychiatry.* 1996; **11**: 705–9.

40 Rodriguez JJ, Ferri CP, Acosta D, *et al.* Prevalence of dementia in Latin America, India, and China: a population-based cross-sectional survey. *Lancet.* 2008; **372**: 464–74.

41 Prince M, Ferri CP, Acosta D, *et al.* The protocols for the 10/66 Dementia Research Group population-based research programme. *BMC Public Health.* 2007; **7**: 165.

42 Kalaria RJ, Maestre GE, Arizaga R, *et al.* Alzheimer's disease and vascular dementia in developing countries: prevalence, management, and risk factors. *Lancet Neurology.* 2008; **7**: 812–26.

43 Ineichen B. Senile dementia in Japan: prevalence and response. *Society for Scientific Medicine.* 1996; 42(2): 169–72.

44 Yoshitake T, Kiyohara Y, Kato I, *et al.* Incidence and risk factors of vascular dementia and Alzheimer's disease in a defined elderly Japanese population: the Hisayama Study. *Neurology.* 1995; **45**: 1161–8.

45 Yamada T, Hattori H, Miura A, *et al.* Prevalence of Alzheimer's disease, vascular dementia and dementia with Lewy bodies in a Japanese population. *Psychiatry and Clinical Neurosciences.* 2001; **55**: 21–5.

46 Osuntokun BO, Adeuja AOG, Schoenberg BS, *et al.* Neurological disorders in Nigerian Africans: a community based study. *Acta Neurologica Scandinavica.* 1987; **75**: 13.

47 Longe AC Osuntokun BO. Prevalence of neurological disorders in Udo, a rural community in Southern Nigeria. *Tropical Geography Medicine.* 1989; **41**: 36–40.

48 Ogunniyi AO, Osuntokun BO, Lekwauwa UB, *et al.* Rarity of dementia (by DSM-III-R) in an urban community in Nigeria. *East African Medical Journal.* 1992; **69**(2): 64–8.

49 Hendrie HC, Osuntokun BO, Hall KS, *et al.* Prevalence of Alzheimer's disease and dementia in two communities: Nigerian Africans and African-Americans. *American Journal of Psychiatry.* 1995; **152**(10): 1485–92.

50 Ogunniyi A, Baiyewu O, Gureje O, *et al.* Epidemiology of dementia in Nigeria: results from the Indianapolis-Ibadan study. *European Journal of Neurology.* 2000; **7**: 485–90.

51 Roorsman B, Hagnell O, Lanke J. Prevalence and incidence of senile and multi-infarct dementia in the Lundby study: A comparison between the time periods 1947–1957 and 1957–1972. *Neuropsychobiology.* 1986; **15**: 122–9.

52 Beard CM, Kokmen E, Offord K, *et al.* Is the prevalence of dementia changing? *Neurology.* 1991; **41**: 1911–14.

53 Kokmen E, Beard CM, O'Brien PC, *et al.* Is the incidence of dementing illness changing? A 25 year time trend study in Rochester, Minnesota (1960–1984). *Neurology.* 1993; **43**: 1887–92.

54 Suh G-H, Shah A. A review of the epidemiological transition in dementia – cross-national comparisons of the indices related to Alzheimer's disease and vascular dementia. *Acta Psychiatrica Scandinavica.* 2001; **104**(1): 4–11.

55 Farrer LA, Cupples LA, Haines JL, *et al.* Effects of age, sex, and ethnicity on the association between apolipoprotein E genotype and Alzheimer disease. A meta-analysis. APOE and Alzheimer Disease Meta Analysis Consortium. *Journal of the American Medical Association.* 1997; **278**: 1349–56.

56 Seshadri S, Drachman DA, Lippa CF. Apolipoprotein E epsilon 4 allele and the lifetime risk of Alzheimer's disease. What physicians know, and what they should know. *Archives of Neurology.* 1995; **52**: 1074–9.

57 Craft S, Teri L, Edland SD, *et al.* Accelerated decline in apolipoprotein E-epsilon4 homozygotes with Alzheimer's disease. *Neurology.* 1998; **51**: 149–53.

58 Mortimer JA, van Duijn CM, Chandra V, *et al.* Head trauma as a risk factor for Alzheimer's disease: a collaborative re-analysis of case-control studies. EURODEM Risk Factors Research Group. *International Journal of Epidemiology.* 1991; **20**(Suppl. 2): 28–35.

59 Launer LJ, Andersen K, Dewey ME, *et al.* Rates and risk factors for dementia and Alzheimer's disease: results from EURODEM pooled analyses. *Neurology.* 1999; **52**(1): 78–84.

60 van Duijn CM, Clayton D, Chandra V, *et al*. Familial aggregation of Alzheimer's disease and related disorders: a collaborative re-analysis of case-control studies. EURODEM Risk Factors Research Group. *International Journal of Epidemiology*. 1991; **20**(Suppl. 2): 13–20.

61 Fratiglioni L, Ahlbom A, Viitanen M, *et al*. Risk factors for late-onset Alzheimer's disease: a population-based, case-control study. *Annals of Neurology*. 1993; **33**: 258–66.

62 Graves AB, White E, Koepsell TD, *et al*. A case-control study of Alzheimer's disease. *Annals of Neurology*. 1990; **28**: 766–74.

63 Doll R. Review: Alzheimer's disease and environmental aluminium. *Age and Ageing*. 1993; **22**: 138–53.

64 Wang HX, Fratiglioni L, Frisoni GB, *et al*. Smoking and the occurrence of Alzheimer's disease: cross-sectional and longitudinal data in a population-based study. *American Journal of Epidemiology*. 1999; **149**: 640–4.

65 Broe GA, Creasey H, Jorm AF, *et al*. Health habits and risk of cognitive impairment and dementia in old age: a prospective study on the effects of exercise, smoking and alcohol consumption. *Australian & New Zealand Journal of Public Health*. 1998; **22**: 621–3.

66 Lindsay J, Laurin D, Verreault R, *et al*. Risk factors for Alzheimer's disease: a prospective analysis from the Canadian Study of Health and Aging. *American Journal of Epidemiology*. 2002; **156**: 445–53.

67 White LR, Petrovitch H, Ross GW, *et al*. Brain aging and midlife tofu consumption. *Journal of the American College of Nutrition*. 2000; **19**: 242–55.

68 Borenstein AR, Mortimer JA, Schofield E, *et al*. Cycad exposure and risk of dementia, MCI, and PDC in the Chamorro population of Guam. *Neurology*. 2007; **68**: 1764–71.

69 Whitmer RA, Gunderson EP, Barrett-Connor E, *et al*. Obesity in middle age and future risk of dementia: a 27 year longitudinal population based study. *British Medical Journal*. 2005; **330**: 261–6.

70 Hofman A, Ott A, Breteler MM, *et al*. Atherosclerosis, apolipoprotein E, and prevalence of dementia and Alzheimer's disease in the Rotterdam Study. *Lancet*. 1997; **349**: 151–4.

71 Katzman R. Education and the prevalence of dementia and Alzheimer's disease. *Neurology*. 1993; **43**: 13–20.

72 Stern Y. Cognitive reserve and Alzheimer's disease. *Alzheimer's Disease and Associated Disorders*. 2006; **20**(Suppl. 2): 69–74.

73 int'Veld BA, Ruitenberg A, Hofman A, *et al*. Nonsteroidal antiinflammatory drugs and the risk of Alzheimer's disease. *New England Journal of Medicine*. 2001; **345**: 1515–21.

74 Jick H, Zornberg GL, Jick, SS, *et al*. Statins and the risk of dementia. *Lancet*. 2000; **356**: 1627–31.

75 McGuinness B, Craig D, Bullock R, *et al*. Statins for the prevention of dementia. *Cochrane Database Syst Rev*. 2009; **2**: CD003160.

76 Shumaker SA, Legault C, Kuller L, *et al*. Conjugated equine estrogens and incidence of probable dementia and mild cognitive impairment in postmenopausal women. *Journal of the American Medical Association*. 2004; **291**: 3005–7.

77 Engelhart MJ, Geerlings MI, Ruitenberg A, *et al*. Dietary intake of antioxidants and risk of Alzheimer disease. *Journal of the American Medical Association*. 2002; **287**: 3223–9.

78 Morris MC, Evans DA, Bienias JL, *et al.* Dietary intake of antioxidant nutrients and the risk of incident Alzheimer disease in a biracial community study. *Journal of the American Medical Association.* 2002; **287**: 3230–7.

79 Burt DB, Zembar MJ, Niederehe G. Depression and memory impairment: a meta-analysis of the association, its pattern, and specificity. *Psychological Bulletin.* 1995; **117**: 285–305.

80 Jorm AF, van Duijn CM, Chandra V, *et al.* Psychiatric history and related exposures as risk factors for Alzheimer's disease: a collaborative re-analysis of case-control studies. EURODEM Risk Factors Research Group. *International Journal of Epidemiology.* 1991; **20**(Suppl. 2): 43–47.

81 Chen P, Ganguli M, Mulsant BH, *et al.* The temporal relationship between depressive symptoms and dementia: a community-based prospective study. *Archives of General Psychiatry.* 1999; **56**: 261–6.

82 Schmand B, Jonker C, Geerlings MI, *et al.* Subjective memory complaints in the elderly: depressive symptoms and future dementia. *British Journal of Psychiatry.* 1997; **171**: 373–6.

83 Prencipe M, Casini AR, Ferretti C. Prevalence of dementia in an elderly rural population: effects of age, sex and education. *Journal of Neurology, Neurosurgery and Psychiatry.* 1996; **60**: 628–33.

84 Pollitt PA. Dementia in old age: an anthropological perspective. *Psychological Medicine.* 1996; **26**: 1061–74.

85 Srinivasan TN, Suresh TR, Rajkumar S. Age estimation in the elderly: relevance to geriatric research in developing countries. *Indian Journal of Psychiatry.* 1993; **35**(1): 58–9.

86 Kua EH, Ko SM, Fones SLC, *et al.* Comorbidity of depression in the elderly: an epidemiological study in a Chinese community. *International Journal of Geriatric Psychiatry.* 1996; **11**: 699–704.

87 Bamforth G, Ineichen B. How to add insult to carers' injuries. *Journal of Dementia Care,* 1996; March/April: 14–15.

CHAPTER 3

Diagnosis and classification

Anna V Richman and Ken CM Wilson

INTRODUCTION

Dementia has been defined as 'an acquired global impairment of intellect, memory and personality ...'.[1] It is usually progressive and irreversible and can be due to a number of different causes. It generally develops gradually. An intercurrent illness or a change in social circumstances may herald its presentation. Dementia of whatever type is usually more common with increasing age. The general criteria for the diagnosis of dementia are:[2]

➤ a decline in memory, most evident in the learning of new information
➤ a decline in other cognitive abilities, characterised by deterioration in judgement and thinking, and in the general processing of information
➤ a decline in emotional control or motivation, or a change in social behaviour
➤ the awareness of the environment is preserved during a period of time sufficiently long to allow the demonstration of the above symptoms
➤ for a confident clinical diagnosis the symptoms should have been present for at least six months.

CAUSES OF DEMENTIA

Once a provisional diagnosis of dementia has been made, the clinician needs to clarify the type of dementia from which the person is suffering. The history of how the impairment has developed, along with appropriate tests and examinations, may help to determine the cause. Dementia was classified traditionally as pre-senile or senile, based on age of onset (before or after 65 years of age respectively). The age of onset may be helpful in deciding on the aetiology, but many of the causes of dementia are found in both age groups, making this traditional approach to classification relatively redundant. Alzheimer's disease is the most common cause of dementia. Other common causes include vascular dementia and Lewy body dementia. Mixed Alzheimer's disease and vascular dementia is not uncommon. These dementias are discussed in more detail later in the chapter. A brief description will now be provided about some of the less common types of dementia.

Frontotemporal dementia

The features of this dementia are an early loss of insight, personality change, hyperorality, non-fluent aphasia and well-preserved spatial orientation. Neurological signs are often absent early in the disease, or are limited to the presence of primitive reflexes. There is an equal incidence in men and women and a high familial incidence. Onset occurs most commonly between the ages of 45 and 65 years and the mean duration of illness is eight years.

Dementia in Pick's disease

This is another progressive dementia commencing in middle age. The general criteria for dementia[2] must be met as well as:
➤ slow onset with steady deterioration
➤ predominance of frontal lobe involvement, evidenced by at least two of: emotional blunting, coarsening of social behaviour, disinhibition, apathy or restlessness, aphasia
➤ early on, memory and parietal lobe functions are relatively preserved.

It may be viewed as a form of frontotemporal dementia with specific pathological features at post-mortem.

Dementia in Creutzfeldt–Jakob disease

The onset is usually in middle or later life. Death occurs within one to two years. The general criteria for dementia must be met[2] along with:
➤ a very rapid progression, with disintegration of virtually all higher cerebral functions
➤ at least one of the following: pyramidal or extrapyramidal or cerebellar symptoms, aphasia, visual impairment.

Dementia in Huntington's disease

Huntington's disease is inherited in an autosomal dominant pattern. It may present with cognitive problems or a movement disorder. Symptoms typically emerge during the third and fourth decades and progression is slow. There are involuntary choreiform movements, as well as slowness of thinking or movement and personality alteration. Apathy or depression may also be present. There must be a family history of the disease.

Dementia in Parkinson's disease

A dementia may develop in the course of established Parkinson's disease. There are no particular distinguishing features for this type of dementia. However, it is important that none of the cognitive impairment is attributable to any medication that the patient may be using.

Dementia in human immunodeficiency virus (HIV) disease

Patients with a diagnosis of HIV infection may develop a dementia in the course of the disease. This may present with a variety of motor and behavioural changes, which are progressive. HIV dementia is very rare in those with asymptomatic HIV infection, affecting less than 1%. In those with symptomatic HIV disease, the prevalence rises to 10–20%.[3]

Alcoholic dementia

Alcohol is known to be neurotoxic, but the existence of 'alcoholic dementia' as a distinct entity is doubtful. Many patients diagnosed with alcoholic dementia actually have Korsakoff's syndrome (an amnesic syndrome, not a dementia). Few studies have looked at people diagnosed with this dementia. One study has estimated that among alcoholics attending an outpatient facility, over 50% of patients aged over 45 years, with a long history of alcohol abuse, will be found to have some degree of cognitive impairment.[4] Most will have minor impairments of memory or concentration etc., but a few will have a dementia. However, the dementia could be a vascular or Alzheimer type dementia. Perhaps the term 'cognitive impairment in association with alcohol' would be more appropriate.

Other causes of dementia

It is important not to forget about other causes of dementia. Some of these are potentially reversible with treatment, but most show a partial response to treatment. These include:

➤ infections, e.g. neurosyphilis
➤ vitamin deficiencies, e.g. B_{12}, folate
➤ endocrine and metabolic disorders, e.g. hypothyroidism
➤ drugs
➤ neoplasms
➤ normal pressure hydrocephalus
➤ subdural haematomas.

Causes of dementia: a summary

➤ *Neurodegenerative*: Alzheimer's; frontotemporal; Lewy body.
➤ *Vascular*: infarction; haemorrhage; vasculitis; Binswanger's disease.

➤ *Endocrine*: thyroid disease; diabetes; Cushing's disease; Addison's disease; parathyroid disease.

➤ *Vitamin deficiencies*: B12; thiamine; nicotinic acid.

➤ *Systemic diseases*: anaemia; respiratory disease; renal disease; hepatic disease.

➤ *Neurological disorders*: head injury; neoplasms; normal pressure hydrocephalus; Parkinson's disease; Huntington's disease.

➤ *Infection*: syphilis; HIV.

Subcortical dementia

Over the last 30 years there has been an emerging view that dementia can also be separated into cortical and subcortical types. The differentiating features of subcortical dementia are said to be a profound slowing of cognition, memory disturbances, frontal executive dysfunction and changes in personality and affect in the absence of aphasias, apraxias and agnosias.[5] Subcortical dementias include those associated with Huntington's disease, Parkinson's disease and HIV. Alzheimer's dementia is the most common cortical dementia. It is well recognised, however, that cortical abnormalities are often found in subcortical diseases and vice versa.

THE IMPORTANCE OF AN ACCURATE DIAGNOSIS

Both the progression of the illness and the treatment will vary according to the cause of the dementia. An accurate diagnosis has become particularly important over the last few years with the introduction of acetylcholinesterase inhibitors for use in Alzheimer's disease. It is also an important issue in the treatment of Lewy body dementia where extreme sensitivity to the side-effects of neuroleptic medication is common. Consequently, the cause of the dementia needs to be clarified so that appropriate medication can be used and the course and prognosis better understood. A thorough history and examination of the patient, including relevant investigations (blood tests, brain scans, etc.), will help to determine the cause, and also help to differentiate it from other common conditions such as depression or delirium, which may present in a similar fashion.

DIAGNOSTIC CRITERIA

Criteria for the diagnosis of dementia vary between different classification systems. The two main classification systems in use are the American Psychiatric Association's *Diagnostic and Statistical Manual of Mental Disorders* (4th ed.) (*DSM-IV*)[6] and the *International Classification of Diseases* (10th ed.) (*ICD-10*).[2] The general criteria for dementia according to *ICD-10* are summarised as follows.

➤ A syndrome due to disease of the brain, usually of a chronic (at least six months) or progressive nature.
➤ There is a disturbance of memory and other higher cortical functions, including thinking, orientation, comprehension, calculation, learning capacity, language and judgement.
➤ Consciousness is not clouded.
➤ The impairments of cognitive function are commonly accompanied by deterioration in emotional control, social behaviour or motivation.

Further criteria may then be applied, specific to each type of dementia.

ALZHEIMER'S DEMENTIA

This is the most common cause of dementia in old age and also occurs in those under 65 years of age. It was first described in 1907 by Alois Alzheimer.[7] He described the case of a woman who died aged 51 years with all the symptoms of dementia. This initially led to Alzheimer's disease being thought of as a disease of younger people. Subsequent work has shown that Alzheimer's disease does occur in both older and younger people.[8]

Clinical features

The disease may go unnoticed at first, and is often mistaken for memory changes associated with normal ageing. Intellectual deterioration is slow to develop, but insight is often lost at an early stage. The disease progresses gradually (*see* Case Study 3.1). The clinical features may be considered in three stages, the patient presenting at any stage.

Case Study 3.1

A 72-year-old lady was seen at home by an old age psychiatrist. The lady herself denied any problems but did admit that her memory was not as good as it used to be. She put this down to old age. Her daughter said that she first noticed her mother's memory problems two years ago and since that time she felt that the problems had got worse. Initially she had difficulty remembering names, telephone numbers, etc., but more recently her mother had got lost on two occasions when she was out doing her shopping. The family had also taken over the preparation of meals after the lady had twice put food in the oven to cook and then forgotten about it, resulting in a smoke-filled kitchen. She had stopped doing the daily crossword and also seemed to have problems dealing with bills and cash. She did not appear to be depressed and was a nonsmoker. She had never been in hospital in her life and was not on any medication. There was no family history of any mental health problems. Recent routine blood tests were all normal and a CT scan of her brain showed no evidence of any vascular problems. On examination she scored poorly on tests of her memory, recall and orientation. A diagnosis of Alzheimer's disease was made and she was referred on to the local memory clinic for further assessment and treatment.

Early stage
This generally lasts from two to three years. The clinical features include:
➤ memory impairment
➤ difficulties performing everyday tasks
➤ impaired concentration
➤ spatial disorientation
➤ disturbances of mood – depression, euphoria or lability of mood
➤ fatigue, anxiety and lack of spontaneity.

Some patients maintain good social competence despite severe cognitive impairment.

Intermediate stage
The above features persist and may deteriorate further. Other features may include:
➤ apraxia and agnosia
➤ deterioration in reading and writing ability
➤ disorientation in time and place (may lead to night-time waking and wandering)
➤ speech problems, e.g. nominal dysphasia
➤ emotional lability and catastrophic reactions (extreme distress and anxiety when unable to complete a task)
➤ extrapyramidal disorders, e.g. increased muscle tone and altered gait
➤ delusions and/or hallucinations.

Late stage
The features of this stage can include:
➤ double incontinence
➤ lack of communication
➤ emaciation
➤ limb contractures
➤ grand mal seizures
➤ primitive reflexes.

The patient often becomes bedridden and death frequently results from a subsequent infection, e.g. a chest infection. Death usually occurs within two to eight years from the onset of the disease. *ICD-10* requires that the general criteria for dementia are met, and that there is no evidence from the history, physical examination or further investigations, e.g. a computed tomography (CT) brain scan, of cerebrovascular disease or any other possible cause of dementia.

There is a large variation in the degree and rate of cognitive decline in patients with Alzheimer's dementia. However, defining the anticipated course of the disease in detail can help patients and their families manage the present and plan for the future. Change can be measured by the rate of decline on cognitive testing and by using staging instruments. Two widely used staging schemes are the Washington University Clinical Dementia Rating (CDR)[9] and the Global Deterioration Scale (GDS).[10]

The GDS divides Alzheimer's disease into seven distinguishable stages. Criteria for many of the stages combine a history (memory problems, self-care, language, gait, etc.) with a mental state examination. The history is mainly obtained from the care-giver. Neither of these scales is sensitive as a measure of short-term change, as movement between stages may take several years. They are used mainly for research or for following patients longitudinally over long time periods.

RISK FACTORS FOR ALZHEIMER'S DISEASE

Dementia is a common cause of disability and dependency in society today. Over the last two decades there has been much interest and research into the risk factors for Alzheimer's dementia. This is an important area because of the potential implications for the prevention of the disease by modifying the risk factors.

Genes as risk factors

In cases of early-onset Alzheimer's disease (starting before 65 years of age), an association has been found with mutations associated with a number of genes, including those found on chromosomes 21, 14 and 1. The link with chromosome 21 is interesting, given that patients with Down's syndrome (trisomy 21) have a much higher incidence of Alzheimer's disease than the general population. However, these mutations account for only 30–50% of all autosomal dominant early-onset cases.[11] A clear autosomal dominant pattern of inheritance is rare in cases starting after 65 years of age. Many genes have been proposed as having importance as risk factors for late-onset cases, but studies of these genes have often not been replicated. There does, however, seem to be an increased risk associated with the possession of one or more copies of the APOE ε4 allele (found on chromosome 19) that codes for apolipoprotein E, variant ε4. Further work has shown that APOE ε4 has its predominant effect by determining when, but not if, a person develops late-onset Alzheimer's disease.[12] It seems though that possession of APOE ε4 is neither necessary, nor sufficient for disease initiation.

Non-genetic risk factors

Non-genetic risk factors are likely to be important in Alzheimer's disease as monozygotic twin concordance rates are only 40%.[13] Whilst much work has been carried out looking at the genetic risk factors, work to determine non-genetic risk factors has been slower.

The incidence and prevalence of Alzheimer's disease doubles every five years after 65 years of age. Age is therefore the single most important risk factor. At all ages, women are at an increased risk of developing Alzheimer's disease (the reverse of the situation with vascular dementia). This may be explained by hormonal factors. Some studies have suggested that oestrogen replacement can prevent or delay the onset of Alzheimer's disease. A 16-year follow-up of nearly 500 women found that hormone replacement therapy led to a 54% reduction in the risk of Alzheimer's disease.[14] A more recent trial was not able to demonstrate any improvement in cognition or disease progression in subjects with Alzheimer's given therapeutic oestrogen.[15]

Poor education has recently been cited as a risk factor for Alzheimer's disease, especially in males.[16] The concept of a protective effect of education has found some support.[17] However, it remains to be seen if it is childhood education that is protective, or whether it is the knowledge acquired over the lifetime.

Boxers experiencing repeated head trauma may develop dementia pugilistica. This is associated with pathological changes similar to those found in Alzheimer's disease. However, recent research has failed to implicate head trauma as a risk factor for Alzheimer's disease.[18] The relationship between Alzheimer's disease and aluminium is also unclear at present. Solvents and other heavy metals have not been shown to be risk factors.

Several studies have shown smoking to be protective against Alzheimer's disease. A confounding factor in these studies may be that those subjects who smoke, die before they reach an age at which Alzheimer's disease is prevalent. Other vascular risk factors such as hypertension and insulin-dependent diabetes have also been associated with Alzheimer's disease.[19]

Conflicting results have come from studies looking at the link between depression and dementia. Some suggest that depression is actually an early manifestation of dementia, whilst in other studies, depressive symptoms have been found to increase the risk of subsequent cognitive decline.[20]

Many studies have reported that the intake of NSAIDs is negatively associated with the risk of developing Alzheimer's disease. These findings should be interpreted with some caution. Patients with Alzheimer's may be less able to complain of pain and therefore receive treatment. These drugs may work by delaying nerve cell damage. This information is summarised in Box 3.1.

Box 3.1   Risk factors for Alzheimer's disease

Increased risk
➤ Increasing age
➤ Female sex

Possible increased risk
➤ Poor education
➤ Head trauma

Possible decreased risk
➤ Smoking
➤ NSAIDs

Evidence unclear at present
➤ Aluminium
➤ Depression

VASCULAR DEMENTIA

The term 'vascular dementia' literally means a dementia due to vascular disease. It encompasses a group of conditions, including multi-infarct dementia, subcortical dementia and Binswanger's subcortical arteriosclerotic encephalopathy. A diagnosis of vascular dementia requires the following *ICD-10* criteria[2] to be met:
➤ the general criteria for dementia
➤ deficits in higher cognitive function are unevenly distributed, with some functions affected and others relatively spared
➤ clinical evidence of focal brain damage, manifest in at least one of the following:
 – unilateral spastic weakness of the limbs
 – unilaterally increased tendon reflexes
 – an extended plantar response
 – pseudobulbar palsy
➤ evidence of a significant cerebrovascular disease, which may reasonably be judged to be aetiologically related to the dementia.

Clinical features

The onset is usually after the age of 65 and may follow a cerebral infarct. It may therefore present more acutely than Alzheimer's disease. Arteriosclerotic changes will often be found in the peripheral and retinal blood vessels, and the patient may well have hypertension. Emotional and personality changes may occur before any memory problems. Cognitive impairment tends to fluctuate in severity once it is established. The disease usually progresses in a stepwise manner, with periods of deterioration that are followed by stable periods or even periods of improvement. These more settled episodes might last for several months in the early stages. Insight may be maintained to a late stage. Other features can include:

➤ minor episodes of cerebral ischaemia (transient ischaemic attacks)
➤ depression (may be a result of retained insight) and anxiety
➤ episodes of emotional lability
➤ epileptic seizures (found in approximately 20% of cases).

The life span averages four to seven years from the time of diagnosis, though it may be much longer. Death may result from ischaemic heart disease, cerebral infarction or renal complications. There are a number of different subtypes of vascular dementia and a brief description of each is given below.

Multi-infarct dementia

This is a type of vascular dementia where the onset is gradual, following a number of ischaemic episodes. Each of these often leads to greater cognitive deficits. It may be caused by large-vessel disease and/or small-vessel disease. It is a predominantly cortical dementia.

Subcortical vascular dementia

In this type of dementia, the cerebral cortex is relatively spared. This contrasts with the clinical picture, which may closely resemble that of Alzheimer's dementia. The general criteria for vascular dementia must be met, as well as a history of hypertension and evidence of vascular disease in the deep white matter of the cerebral hemispheres, with preservation of the cerebral cortex.

Binswanger's disease

This is also known as progressive small-vessel disease or subcortical arteriosclerotic encephalopathy. It is a rare form of vascular dementia, first described by Binswanger in 1894.[21] Dementia may dominate the clinical picture but there may be concomitant physical problems, e.g. dysarthria and gait disorders. It is classically a slowly progressive dementia.

Cerebral autosomal dominant arteriopathy with subcortical infarcts and leukoencephalopthy (CADASIL)

A rare familial form of vascular dementia. Patients usually present in their 40s with recurrent strokes. Quite often there is a history of migraine and many patients go on to develop a subcortical dementia and pseudobulbar palsy.

Other rare causes of vascular dementia

Cerebral vasculitis may cause repeated infarcts, and these may result in a dementia. The vasculitis usually involves many organs, resulting in other systemic features, e.g. systemic lupus erythematosus. Cognitive problems may also be noted after cerebral and extracerebral haemorrhages, often as a residual problem. Dementia may also occur as a result of multiple infarcts occurring during hypotensive crises, and as a result of chronic subdural haematomas.

THE HACHINSKI SCORE

Hachinski developed a scoring system which has been widely used as a guide to help clinicians distinguish between vascular dementia and Alzheimer's dementia.[22] The features are weighted as shown in Box 3.2. The scores of all features present are added together to give a total score, and a total score above six suggests a vascular dementia.

Box 3.2   The Hachinski ischaemia score

Abrupt onset	2
Stepwise deterioration	1
Fluctuating course	2
Nocturnal confusion	1
Relative preservation of personality	1
Depression	1
Somatic complaints	1
Emotional incontinence	1
History of hypertension	1
History of strokes	2
Atherosclerosis	2
Focal neurological symptoms	2
Focal neurological signs	2

DIFFERENTIATING BETWEEN VASCULAR DEMENTIA AND ALZHEIMER'S DEMENTIA

Characteristically, Alzheimer's disease has an insidious onset and progresses slowly without any evidence of focal brain damage. In contrast, vascular dementia tends to present more acutely and progress in a stepwise manner. Findings compatible with ischaemic brain changes are also present. At times it is therefore clearly possible to differentiate the two types of dementia. At other times though, it can be quite the opposite. Brain imaging techniques may be used to help in the diagnosis, e.g. to identify cerebral infarcts. As mentioned above, the Hachinski score is also used to assist in the diagnosis. However, sometimes the diagnosis can only be confirmed at post-mortem. It must also be remembered that a mixed vascular and Alzheimer's dementia is not uncommon.[23]

RISK FACTORS FOR VASCULAR DEMENTIA

The incidence of vascular dementia in men and women is almost equal, but it is slightly more common in men. There is considerable evidence to suggest that raised blood pressure earlier in life is a risk factor for dementia in later life. Research has shown that hypertension is the most important remedial risk factor for stroke and vascular dementia.[24] Work is ongoing at present to assess the effectiveness of antihypertensives in vascular dementia. Advancing age is a risk factor for stroke, and therefore also for vascular dementia.

Several studies have reported an increased incidence of dementia after strokes. However, not all cases of vascular dementia can be explained by the sequelae of stroke, ischaemia or hypoxia.

Cerebral white matter lesions are seen more frequently in patients with vascular dementia than in normal elderly subjects or patients with other dementias.

They have been shown to be predictors of post-stroke dementia.[25] A history of myocardial infarction is also a risk factor for vascular dementia, as are atrial fibrillation, rheumatic valvular disease and carotid artery stenosis. Diabetes is a risk factor for vascular disease as it is associated with a reduction in cerebral perfusion, which may result in infarctions.[26]

Raised levels of low-density lipoproteins, in particular, have been shown to be a risk factor for the development of dementia with stroke. This relationship has not been found with Alzheimer's disease.[27]

Smoking has been shown to be a risk factor for vascular dementia by some,[28] but these results have not always been replicated. As with Alzheimer's dementia, a possible explanation could be that those who smoke have reduced life spans, and may die before developing a dementia. Many studies have shown an increased risk of vascular dementia in people with a history of alcohol misuse,[24] but not all studies have found this.[28]

There are many rare genetic disorders that are associated with stroke and subsequent vascular dementia. An increased risk of stroke or coronary heart disease has also been shown in patients with the APOE polymorphism. As previously stated, this is a risk factor for Alzheimer's disease. It is important to note here that many patients with Alzheimer's disease also have vascular changes, and one-fifth have been shown to have vascular lesions.[24] It is likely that the co-existing vascular problems in these patients will contribute to their cognitive decline.

Poor formal education has been associated with an increased risk of vascular dementia,[24] as have psychological stress in early life and 'blue-collar' occupations.[29] The Canadian Study of Health and Ageing showed elevated odds ratios for vascular dementia in people who had occupational exposure to pesticides, fertilisers, liquid plastics and rubbers.[24] This information is summarised in Box 3.3.

Box 3.3   Risk factors for vascular dementia

Increased risk
➤ Male sex
➤ Increasing age
➤ Hypertension
➤ Diabetes mellitus
➤ Previous stroke
➤ Cardiovascular disease
➤ High levels of low-density lipoproteins

Possible increased risk
➤ Smoking
➤ Alcohol misuse
➤ Poor education
➤ 'Blue collar' occupations
➤ Psychological stress in early life
➤ Previous exposure to pesticides, fertilisers, etc.

In order to reduce the risk of both stroke and vascular dementia, it is important that these risk factors are identified and treated as early as possible. Some cases of vascular dementia could be prevented (*see* Case Study 3.2).

Since this chapter was drafted for the first edition, the concept of vascular cognitive impairment (VCI) has gained currency.[30] This emphasises that VCI often *precedes* the development of frank dementia with predominant cortical features. VCI (at least in its early stages) is predominantly a subcortical phenomenon, with early impairment of frontal lobe function. Early detection may facilitate preventive measures to slow or stop the development of frank dementia. In VCI a history of stroke is missing in more than half the cases, and focal signs are also often missing. The classical 'patchy' function of vascular dementia (usually only dominant when the dementia is due to a limited number of large infarcts) is not found in VCI. As yet there are no validated diagnostic criteria for VCI though guidelines have been published.[31] It remains to be seen whether and how this concept (along with Lewy body dementia) will find its way into the new *ICD-11* system expected in 2015.

Case Study 3.2

A 78-year-old gentleman went to see his GP with his wife. Over the last few months he had noticed that he had become increasingly forgetful, and his wife confirmed this. He was concerned that he may have Alzheimer's disease. The problems seemed to come on quite suddenly and since that time he reported episodes when he felt that his memory was awful, but other times when it was fairly good. He had mislaid items around the house and had put teabags in the kettle on a few occasions when making a cup of tea. His wife had also had to help him with their finances, as he no longer felt able to do this himself. He often had difficulty remembering the names of his children. There was no past psychiatric history but the patient was on treatment for hypertension and angina. He also smoked 20 cigarettes a day and had done so for 50 years. He did have some problems with his memory and concentration when the GP tested him. The GP requested a CT scan, which showed some brain atrophy and evidence of old infarctions. A diagnosis of a vascular dementia was made by the GP.

LEWY BODY DEMENTIA

Lewy bodies are the pathological hallmark of Parkinson's disease. However, they have also been found to occur in the cerebral cortex in association with dementia. Lewy body dementia is a common form of dementia in old age. Many patients with Lewy body dementia also show some Alzheimer-type changes, and minor vascular disease occurs in approximately 30%, i.e. mixed pathological changes are usually seen.[32]

Clinical features

Dementia is usually the presenting feature. However, patients may present with Parkinsonism, psychiatric disorder in the absence of dementia, falls, orthostatic hypotension or transient disturbances of consciousness.[33] The age at onset ranges from 50 to 83 years. Survival time from diagnosis is similar to that for Alzheimer's disease, but some patients do show a rapid progression of symptoms and death may occur within one to two years in these cases. The cognitive function seems to decline at a similar rate to that in Alzheimer's disease. It is slightly more common in men than women. Clinical features include:
➤ fluctuation in cognitive performance and level of consciousness (usually evident day to day), with pronounced variations in attention and alertness
➤ visual hallucinations (reported by approximately two-thirds of patients) – these are usually well formed and detailed

➤ depression (occurs in 40%)
➤ Parkinsonism (occurs in up to 70% of patients, e.g. bradykinesia, limb rigidity and gait disturbances)
➤ repeated falls and syncope.

Other features that may support the diagnosis are sensitivity to neuroleptic medication (found in up to 50% of patients), systematised delusions and hallucinations in other modalities. Lewy body dementia is a fairly new concept and is not defined within *ICD-10*, but consensus criteria for the clinical diagnosis of probable and possible dementia with Lewy bodies have been put forward.[34] These include the features mentioned above and also state that a diagnosis of Lewy body dementia is less likely in the presence of stroke disease, or if there is evidence of any physical illness or other brain disorder which could account for the clinical picture. The diagnostic accuracy has not yet been established outside of specialist research settings and this is an area for further work. There is also a grey area between the diagnoses of Lewy body dementia and Parkinson's disease with dementia or psychosis. Should these all be classified as a 'Lewy body disease spectrum' or should they remain as separate categories? The debate is ongoing.

There is obviously much more work to be done within the field of Lewy body dementia, especially with regard to establishing diagnostic accuracy in the community and defining aetiological factors. Research is also currently ongoing to find effective treatments for Lewy body dementia.

DEPRESSIVE PSEUDODEMENTIA
An elderly person may present with reduced interests, psychomotor retardation, slowed thinking and concentration, poor short-term memory and disorientation. This readily mimics dementia when actually there is an underlying depression, hence the term depressive pseudodementia. However, it must be remembered that depression frequently occurs in the early stages of dementia, so the diagnosis may be difficult. When the situation is unclear, a careful history and mental state should help to differentiate the two. Points to consider are as follows.
➤ Onset – more likely to be acute in depression and insidious in dementia.
➤ Memory decline prior to the current episode – less likely in depression than in dementia.
➤ Observations from a close family member.
➤ Is the patient distressed by the situation? Patients with depression will often complain of their difficulties, unlike patients with dementia.
➤ Responses to questions – a tendency in depressed patients to reply, 'Don't know', whereas a patient with dementia may confabulate or make excuses for not knowing.

➤ Any family history of depression or dementia?
➤ Are symptoms of depression present?
➤ Performance on cognitive function tests – may be inconsistent in depression, where inattention is often the main problem and dysphasia and dyspraxia will be absent.

These points may help when trying to differentiate between depression and dementia.

DELIRIUM SUPERIMPOSED ON DEMENTIA

Patients with dementia may also present as acutely confused at times. This is often described as an acute on chronic confusion or as a delirium superimposed on dementia. The definition of delirium in *ICD-10*[2] is as follows:
➤ there is clouding of consciousness
➤ disturbance of cognition is manifest by impairment of immediate recall and recent memory (with relatively intact remote memory), and also disorientation in time, place or person
➤ At least one of:
  – rapid unpredictable shifts from hypoactivity to hyperactivity
  – increased reaction time
  – increased or decreased flow of speech
  – enhanced startle reaction
➤ disturbance of sleep or the sleep–wake cycle, causing insomnia and/ or nocturnal worsening of symptoms and/or disturbing dreams and nightmares
➤ symptoms have a rapid onset and fluctuate over the course of the day
➤ obvious evidence of an underlying cerebral or systemic disease that can be presumed to be responsible for the clinical manifestations.

Almost any acute illness can cause a delirium in an elderly person. The most common causes are urinary tract infections, chest infections, cardiac failure and iatrogenic causes.

Dementia is a risk factor for delirium; indeed, it has been identified as one of three major risk factors for delirium.[35] Other predisposing factors include:[36]
➤ ageing or disease of the brain
➤ impairment of vision and hearing
➤ reduced synthesis of neurotransmitters
➤ changes in pharmacokinetics and dynamics of drugs
➤ high prevalence of chronic diseases
➤ high susceptibility to acute diseases
➤ reduced capacity for homeostatic regulation.

A thorough history with a mental state examination, a physical examination and appropriate investigations should help to determine the cause. The appropriate specific treatment can then be administered, along with supportive care. This is most often undertaken in a general hospital.

As this book goes to press, new research diagnostic criteria have been proposed for Alzheimer's disease that define a pre-symptomatic stage and rely more heavily on sophisticated neuroimaging (see Chapter 4 and www.alz.org/research/diagnostic_criteria for more information on the neuroimaging techniques and research diagnostic criteria respectively).

Key points

➤ Dementia is a syndrome with a number of different causes.

➤ It is usually more common with increasing age, progressive and irreversible.

➤ The most common types of dementia are Alzheimer's disease, vascular dementia and Lewy body dementia.

➤ Defining the cause of the dementia will inform decisions on treatment and prognosis.

➤ Diagnostic criteria for dementia can be found in *DSM-IV* and *ICD-10*.

➤ A full history, mental state examination, physical examination and further investigations, e.g. blood tests and CT scans, should help to clarify the cause of the dementia.

➤ Alzheimer's disease is the most common cause of dementia. It tends to progress gradually through three clinical stages.

➤ Whilst an autosomal dominant pattern has been described in several cases of Alzheimer's disease starting before 65 years of age, this is extremely rare in those cases starting after 65 years.

➤ Several non-genetic risk factors for Alzheimer's disease have been proposed.

➤ Vascular dementia may present acutely and characteristically progresses in a stepwise manner.

➤ Many of the risk factors for vascular dementia are the same as those for cardiovascular disease. Early identification and treatment of these risk factors could therefore potentially prevent some cases of vascular dementia.

➤ Lewy body dementia has been described more recently and consensus criteria for its diagnosis have been proposed which describe the clinical features.

> ➤ Mixed patterns of dementia, such as mixed Alzheimer's and vascular dementia, are not uncommon.
> ➤ Depressive pseudodementia and delirium superimposed on dementia should be considered when a patient presents with a possible diagnosis of dementia.

REFERENCES

1 Lishman WA. *Organic Psychiatry*. Oxford: Blackwell Science; 1987.
2 World Health Organization. *The ICD-10 Classification of Mental and Behavioural Disorders: clinical descriptions and diagnostic guidelines*. Geneva: WHO; 1992.
3 McArthur JC, Hoover DR, Bacellar H, *et al.* Dementia in AIDS patients: incidence and risk factors. *Neurology*. 1993; **43**: 2245–52.
4 Edwards G. *The Treatment of Drinking Problems*. London: Grant McIntyre; 1982.
5 Cummings JL. Subcortical dementia. Neuropsychology, neuropsychiatry and pathophysiology. *British Journal of Psychiatry*. 1986; **149**: 682–97.
6 American Psychiatric Association. *Diagnostic and Statistical Manual of Mental Disorders*. 4th ed. Washington DC: APA; 1994.
7 Alzheimer A. Uber eine eigenartige Erkrankung der Hirnrinde. *Allgemeine Zeitschrift fur Psychiatrie und Psychisch-Gerichtlich Medizin*. 1907; **64**: 146–8.
8 Gao S, Hendrie HC, Hall KS, *et al.* The relationships between age, sex and the incidence of dementia and Alzheimer disease: a meta-analysis. *Archives of General Psychiatry*. 1998; **55**: 809–15.
9 Hughes CP, Berg L, Danziger W, *et al.* A new clinical scale for the staging of dementia. *British Journal of Psychiatry*. 1982; **140**: 566–72.
10 Reisberg B, Ferris S, De Leon MJ, *et al.* The Global Deterioration Scale (GDS): an instrument for the assessment of primary degenerative dementia. *American Journal of Psychiatry*. 1982; **139**: 1136–9.
11 Cruts M, van Duijn CM, Backhovens H, *et al.* Estimation of the genetic contribution of presenilin-1 and -2 mutations in a population based study of presenile Alzheimer's disease. *Human Molecular Genetics*. 1998; **7**: 43–51.
12 Meyer MR, Tschanz JT, Norton MC, *et al.* APOE genotype predicts when – not whether – one is predisposed to develop Alzheimer's disease. *Nature Genetics*. 1998; **19**: 321–2.
13 Pericak-Vance MA, Haines JL. Genetic susceptibility to Alzheimer's disease. *Trends in Genetics*. 1995; **11**: 504–8.
14 Kawas C, Resnick S, Morrison A, *et al.* A prospective study of estrogen replacement therapy and the risk of developing Alzheimer's disease: the Baltimore Longitudinal Study of Aging. *Neurology*. 1997; **48**: 1517–21.
15 Mulnard RA, Cotman CW, Kawas C, *et al.* Estrogen replacement therapy for treatment of mild to moderate Alzheimer's disease: a randomised controlled trial. Alzheimer's Disease Cooperative Study. *Journal of the American Medical Association*. 2000; **283**: 1007–15.
16 Ott A, van Rossum CT, van Harskamp F, *et al.* Education and the incidence of

dementia in a large population-based study: the Rotterdam Study. *Neurology.* 1999; **52**: 663–6.

17 Orrell M, Sahakian B. Education and dementia. *British Medical Journal.* 1995; **310**: 951–2.

18 Launer LJ, Andersen K, Dewey ME, *et al.* Rates and risk factors for dementia and Alzheimer's disease: results from EURODEM pooled analyses. EURODEM Incidence Research Group and Work Groups – European studies of dementia. *Neurology.* 1999; **52**: 78–84.

19 Stewart R, Prince M, Mann A. Vascular risk factors and Alzheimer's disease. *Australian & New Zealand Journal of Psychiatry.* 1999; **33**: 809–13.

20 Yaffe K, Blackwell T, Gore R. *et al.* Depressive symptoms and cognitive decline in nondemented elderly women: a prospective study. *Archives of General Psychiatry.* 1999; **56**: 425–30.

21 Binswanger O. Die Abgrenzung der allgemeinen progressiven paralyse. *Berliner klinische Wochenshrift.* 1984; **31**: 1137–9.

22 Hachinski VC, Lliff LD, Kilhka M, *et al.* Cerebral blood flow in dementia. *Archives of Neurology.* 1975; **32**: 632–7.

23 Jellinger K, Danielczyk W, Fischer P, *et al.* Clinicopathological analysis of dementia disorders in the elderly. *Journal of Neurological Sciences.* 1990; **95**: 239–58.

24 Lindsay J, Hebert R, Rockwood K. The Canadian Study of Health and Aging: risk factors for vascular dementia. *Stroke.* 1997; **28**: 526–30.

25 Miyos S, Takano A, Teramoto J, *et al.* Leukoariosis in relation to prognosis for patients with lacunar infarction. *Stroke.* 1992; **233**: 1434–8.

26 Desmond DW, Tatemichi TK, Paik M, *et al.* Risk factors for cerebrovascular disease as correlates of cognitive function in a stroke-free cohort. *Archives of Neurology.* 1993; **50**: 162–6.

27 Moroney JT, Tang MX, Bergkind L, *et al.* Low-density lipoprotein cholesterol and the risk of dementia with stroke. *Journal of the American Medical Association.* 1999; **282**: 254–60.

28 Meyer JS, McClintik K, Rogers RL, *et al.* Aetiological considerations and risk factors for multi-infarct dementia. *Journal of Neurology and Neurosurgical Psychiatry.* 1988; **51**: 1489–97.

29 Peerson G, Skoog I. A prospective population study of psychosocial risk factors for late-onset dementia. *International Journal of Geriatric Psychiatry.* 1996; **11**: 15–22.

30 Bowler JV. Modern concept of vascular cognitive impairment. *British Medical Bulletin.* 2007; **83**: 291–305.

31 Hachinski V, Iadecola C, Peterson RC, *et al.* National Institute of Neurological Disorders and Stroke – Canadian stroke network vascular cognitive impairment harmonisation standards. *Stroke.* 2006; **37**: 2220–41.

32 Holmes C, Cairns N, Lantos P, *et al.* Validity of current clinical criteria for Alzheimer's disease, vascular dementia and dementia with Lewy bodies. *British Journal of Psychiatry.* 1999; **174**: 45–50.

33 McKeith IG, Perry RH, Fairbairn AF, *et al.* Operational criteria for senile dementia of Lewy body type (SDLT). *Psychological Medicine.* 1992; **22**: 911–22.

34 McKeith IG, Galasko D, Kosaka K, *et al.* Consensus guidelines for the clinical and pathologic diagnosis of dementia with Lewy bodies (DLB): report of the consortium on DLB international workshop. *Neurology.* 1996; **47**: 1113–24.

35 O'Keefe S, Lavan J. Predicting delirium in elderly patients: development and validation of a risk-stratification model. *Age and Ageing*. 1996; **25**: 317–21.

36 Lipowski ZJ. Delirium (acute confusional states). *Journal of the American Geriatrics Society*. 1987; **258**: 1789–92.

CHAPTER 4

Early detection of dementia

Sonja Krüger, Miguel A Bertoni and Stephen Curran

INTRODUCTION

Dementia is one of the most significant health and social care challenges of this century. It is a clinical syndrome of acquired cognitive impairment produced by brain dysfunction. It is a common disorder in older adults, involving as many as 10% of those over 65 years. Alzheimer's disease (AD) is the most common cause of dementia, and its prevalence doubles every five years after the age of 65 years and reaches nearly 50% after the age of 85 years. According to the World Health Organization, there are currently an estimated 20 million of people with AD worldwide. There is no known cure for AD but the anticholinesterase treatments, donepezil (Aricept), rivastigmine (Exelon) and galantamine (Reminyl), together with the partial N-methyl-D-asparate (NMDA) inhibitor, memantine (Ebixa) which acts on glutamate pathways, often ameliorate the condition.

In AD and other forms of dementia, irreversible brain damage usually occurs before clinical symptoms become apparent. The sooner anti-dementia drugs can be given to patients, the greater the potential clinical benefit. This has led to a clinical and ethical drive to try to detect AD at an early stage, ideally before memory disturbance or other symptoms become apparent. There is therefore a pressing need for an easy-to-use and inexpensive means of screening people at risk of developing AD which would help to diagnose AD at an early stage. Other forms of dementia also need to be identified early so that further decline can be halted or symptoms reversed.

Tests which are used as screening instruments are generally quick and easy to use and help to identify potential cases of AD. These cases can then be examined in greater detail using a variety of techniques to establish the diagnosis. In addition, a number of tests may be potentially useful as screening instruments, such as neuro-imaging techniques. Cost or practical considerations might still hamper their day-to-day use in the clinical setting.

Clinical methods currently remain the gold standard for the ante-mortem diagnosis of dementia and AD. In addition, clinical and pathological classifications will remain the backbone of interpreting these methods and in advancing our understanding of the complex interplay between genotype and phenotype.

RISKS AND BENEFITS OF EARLY DETECTION

The early detection of dementia is important for a number of reasons. Firstly, early diagnosis will give patients an opportunity to discuss their symptoms, treatment options and prognosis and make informed choices about their future. Patients will be able to plan for the future, make their wishes known about residential care and other issues, such as setting-up an enduring power of attorney. Families can also be supported at a much earlier stage and crises can be minimised or avoided. Patients with reversible causes for their cognitive impairment, e.g. vitamin B_{12} deficiency, can be treated (*see* Box 4.2 on page 61) and symptoms frequently reversed. Patients with vascular dementia can stabilise their symptoms in part by improving their physical health and a number of lifestyle changes such as stopping smoking, eating a healthier diet, doing more exercise. In addition, lifestyle changes geared to improvements in cardiovascular health could also impact on the onset AD, since risk factors for cerebrovascular disease are also risk factors for dementia, including AD.[1] Hence, interventions that modify vascular risk factors might also be able to delay the onset of AD or slow its rate of progression. In addition, drugs for the treatment of AD are more likely to be effective if they are given early, although paradoxically the effects at this stage may be less obvious.[2] From the research point of view, early and accurate detection and diagnosis is important in allowing assessment of the efficacy of interventions at a stage when they are likely to be most effective.

Early detection is therefore important as it:
➤ gives patients a greater say in their future care
➤ helps patients and their families to plan for the future
➤ may enhance the effectiveness of medication
➤ enables research into the efficacy of early intervention.

At least for a subset of patients, the clinical diagnosis of mild cognitive impairment (MCI) may represent an intermediate stage between normal ageing and dementia. Nevertheless, the patterns of transition of cognitive states between normal cognitive ageing and MCI to dementia are not well established. In a recent study by Forlenza and colleagues at the Sao Paolo University in Brazil, the pattern of transitions between cognitive states in patients with MCI and healthy controls, prior to the conversion to dementia, was addressed.[3] One hundred and thirty-nine subjects (78% women, mean age 68.5 +/- 6.1 years;

mean educational level 11.7 +/− 5.4 years) were consecutively assessed in a memory clinic with a standardised clinical and neuropsychological protocol, and classified as cognitively healthy (normal controls) or with MCI (including subtypes) at baseline. These subjects underwent annual reassessments (mean duration of follow-up 2.7 +/− 1.1 years), in which cognitive state was ascertained independently of prior diagnoses. The transitions from one cognitive state to another varied substantially between MCI subtypes. Single-domain MCI (amnestic and non-amnestic) more frequently returned to normal cognitive state upon follow-up (22.5% and 21%, respectively). Among subjects who progressed to AD, the most common diagnosis immediately prior to conversion was multiple-domain MCI (85%). The study concluded that the presence of more severe and widespread cognitive deficits, as indicated by the group of multiple-domain amnestic MCI, may be a better predictor of AD than single-domain amnestic or non-amnestic deficits. These higher-risk individuals could probably be the best candidates for the development of preventive strategies and early treatment for the disease.

As can be predicted, not all the consequences of early detection are necessarily positive. The diagnosis will be stressful for patients and carers and because the natural history of dementia is well known, it can be an alarming diagnosis and can result in a range of psychological reactions, including 'shock and bewilderment' initially, followed by a range of emotions such as anger, depression and denial. However a particular patient and their family copes with the diagnosis, it is nearly always stressful and it has a dramatic impact on their lives and future plans. If the diagnosis subsequently turns out to be wrong, the consequences can be devastating and patients and their families will feel very angry. If possible pre- and post-diagnostic counselling should be available, but this is rarely the case. This will become more of a priority if the 'Holy Grail' of a blood test for AD that can predict the clinical onset of the disease becomes a reality. Some recent promising work has demonstrated an association of plasma clusterin concentration with severity, pathology and progression of AD.[4]

In the early stages, overlap with healthy ageing and depression is common and a balance needs to be struck between early diagnosis and getting the diagnosis correct. There is currently no diagnostic test for many of the different kinds of dementia, and AD in particular, but as the condition progresses accurate diagnosis usually becomes easier.

CHARACTERISTICS OF DIAGNOSTIC AND SCREENING TESTS

There is considerable overlap between screening and diagnostic tests and to some extent they have similar characteristics. A *screening* instrument needs to be relatively simple to use. It is usually administered to large groups of people and those patients identified are then subjected to more intensive investigation. Screening instruments have a number of desirable characteristics, some of which are practical in nature, some cost-related and some methodological. Screening instruments should be easy to administer for both the tester and patient; they should be relatively quick, safe and cheap to administer and should not cause undue anxiety for the patient. They should also be portable and require minimal training. They should be valid (measure what the test is supposed to measure such as cognitive function) and reliable. The latter requirement can be split into test–retest reliability (are the results the same on two separate occasions?) and inter-rater reliability (are the results the same when the test is administered by two different people?). Screening instruments usually identify patients who are more likely to have a disorder but require further investigation, e.g. patients who score poorly on the Mini-Mental State Examination (MMSE) test – which might be due to a number of factors. Further questioning and examination might lead to a diagnosis of AD, but the MMSE is not a diagnostic test – what is detected (cognitive impairment) is not specific to dementia. For this reason, additional assessment is needed to make the diagnosis. In this sense most of the so-called 'diagnostic' tests are really screening tests.

Tests should also be sensitive and specific. The sensitivity is the ability of the test to *correctly detect the condition*, and is the proportion of people with the condition who test positive. The specificity is the ability of the test to *correctly identify subjects who do not have the condition*, and is the proportion of people without the condition who test negative. The ideal test should correctly identify all subjects with the condition, as well as all subjects without the condition, and would have a sensitivity and specificity both equal to 100%. Tests that make 'mistakes' are less than ideal and miss the condition in some subjects who do have it and/or identify the condition in some subjects who do not have it. The concept of sensitivity and specificity is summarised in Table 4.1. The sensitivity is $a/(a+c)$ whereas the specificity is $d/(b+d)$.[5] Some of the other commonly used terms include *positive predictive value* (PPV) (if the test is positive, the PPV is the probability that the patient has the condition $a/(a+b)$) and *negative predictive value* (NPP) (if the test is negative, the NPP is the probability that the patient does not have the condition $d/(c+d)$).

Table 4.1 Table for calculating sensitivity and specificity

	Disease present	*Disease absent*
Test positive	a	b
Test negative	c	d

a = true positives, b = false positives, c = false negatives and d = true negatives. In an ideal test, b = c = 0.

Potential screening tests can be classified into a number of groups, including clinical assessment, rating scales, other psychometric tests, neuroimaging techniques, biochemical tests, biopsy and genetic tests. Although there is considerable overlap between screening and diagnostic tests, these have been separated for convenience. Screening tests are usually not diagnostic but are used to identify patients at high risk of having a particular condition, such as AD. These patients can then undergo a fuller diagnostic evaluation. The situation is further confused by simple tests that can be used in the community and those that tend either to be confined to specialist centres or are not widely available because they are still undergoing evaluation.

DIAGNOSTIC TESTS

Clinical assessment

Clinical assessment is an important part of the diagnostic process and should include a detailed history, a mental state examination, a physical examination and information should be obtained from other sources, especially carers. The nature of the memory impairment as well as its course, duration and associated features, such as focal signs, should be evaluated. Previous psychiatric history, family history of memory impairment and current medication can also be very helpful. In addition, many drugs, especially psychiatric drugs, can cause confusion and memory impairment. The patient's medical history is also important as this might point to a specific cause – examples include cerebrovascular disease, head injury and vitamin B_{12} deficiency. Additional aspects of the history that should be asked about include previous occupation, activities of daily living, the presence of psychiatric symptoms such as depression and psychotic symptoms and any carer stress. This information combined with further investigations will help to establish the diagnosis. As well as identifying a specific cause of the dementia they will also identify any potentially reversible cause for the dementia (*see* Box 4.2 on page 61) and any psychiatric syndromes such as depression, anxiety or psychotic phenomena that will require treatment in their own right. Attention to these will improve not only the quality of life for patients with cognitive impairment but also in some cases reduce their mortality, particularly in the case of depression.

The current clinical criteria for diagnosis of AD are focused mostly on cognitive deficits produced by dysfunction of hippocampal and high-order neocortical areas, whereas non-cognitive, behavioural and psychological symptoms of dementia, such as disturbances in mood, emotion, appetite and wake–sleep cycle, confusion, agitation and depression, have been less considered. The early occurrence of these symptoms suggests brainstem involvement, and more specifically of the serotonergic nuclei.[6] Several recent reports have drawn attention to the possibility of selective and early involvement of raphe nuclei, particularly the dorsal raphe nucleus (DRN), in the pathogenesis of AD. Based on these findings of differential susceptibility and anatomical connectivity, a novel pathogenetic scheme of AD progression is now proposed. Although the precise mechanisms of neurofibrillary degeneration still await elucidation, researchers speculate that cumulative oxidative damage may be the main cause of DRN alterations, as age is the main risk factor for sporadic AD. Within such a framework, beta-amyloid production is considered only as one of the factors (although a significant one in familial cases) that promotes molecular series of events underlying AD-related neuropathological changes.

Dubois and colleagues recently proposed that it is possible to recognise the pre-dementia stage of AD by adopting a multidimensional approach, identifying:

➤ a specific amnestic disorder of the hippocampal type
➤ the atrophy of medial temporal structures – specifically the hippocampus
➤ the specific profile of cerebrospinal fluid biomarkers or of metabolic neuroimaging changes.

An international working group was convened to discuss the opportunity to develop a diagnostic framework for AD that would include the prodromal stages. At the end of this consensus meeting it was concluded that it was possible to recognise AD at the prodromal, pre-dementia stage with the use of specific memory tests, biomarkers and neuroimaging investigations. There was no longer a reason to limit the diagnosis of AD to patients who reached the threshold of full-blown dementia. Accordingly, it was decided that new criteria be proposed that would apply both in the early stages and across the full spectrum of the illness.[7] These criteria are set out in Box 4.1 below.

To satisfy criterion A, memory symptoms must start gradually and show progressive decline over at least six months. Particular attention should be paid to intra-individual decline, which improves the identification of those individuals with prodromal AD. The proposed criteria emphasise the specificity of memory changes of AD and the need to use specific memory tests. It is noteworthy that most of the current memory tests do not record whether items to be recalled have been truly registered. Effective encoding of information should be controlled in order to exclude memory deficit related to anxiety, depression, frontal dysfunction or any other functional disorder. In the same way, identification of AD can be improved by using semantic cueing that facilitates the retrieval of stored information in aged healthy people or in patients with subcorticofrontal dysfunction. Reduced benefit of cueing at recall reliably identifies prodromal AD. Episodic memory impairment is proposed as a core feature of AD. It can be isolated or associated with other cognitive changes at the onset of AD or as AD advances. Compare this section with the outline in Chapter 6. The present section refers more to 'cutting-edge' work whereas that

Box 4.1   Diagnostic criteria for Alzheimer's disease[7]

Probable AD: A plus one or more supportive features B, C or D
Core diagnostic criteria
A   Presence of an early and significant episodic memory impairment
that includes the following features:
- ➤ Gradual progressive change in memory function reported by the
patient or informant over more than six months.
- ➤ Objective evidence of significantly impaired episodic memory
on testing. This generally consists of memory performance that
does not improve significantly with cueing or recognition testing
and after effective encoding of information has been previously
controlled.
- ➤ The episodic memory impairment can be isolated or associated
with other cognitive changes at the onset of AD or as AD advances.
Supportive features
B   Presence of MTL atrophy:
Volume loss of hippocampl, entorhinal cortex or amygdale
evidenced on MRI with:
- ➤ qualitative ratings using visual scoring (referenced to well
characterised population with age norms) or quantitative
volumetry of regions of interest (referenced to well characterised
populations with age norms).
C   Abnormal CSF biomarkers:
- ➤ decreased Aβ 1–42 and/or increased total tau and/or increased
phosphor-tau
- ➤ other well validated markers to be discovered in the future.
D   Specific pattern in functional neuroimaging with PET:
- ➤ reduced glucose metabolism in bilateral temporal parietal
regions
- ➤ other well validated ligands, including those that will emerge
such as PiB or FDDNP.
Exclusion criteria
History:
- ➤ sudden onset
- ➤ early occurrence of the following symptoms – gait disturbances,
seizures, behavioural changes.
Clinical features:
- ➤ focal neurological features including hemiparesis, sensory loss,
visual field deficits
- ➤ early extrapyramidal signs.

Other medical conditions severe enough to account for memory and related symptoms:

➤ non-AD dementia

➤ major depression

➤ cerebrovascular disease

➤ toxic and metabolic abnormalities, all of which may require specific investigation

➤ MRI FLAIR or T2 signal abnormalities in the MTL that are consistent with infectious or vascular insults.

AD – Alzheimer's disease

MTL – medial temporal lobe

CSF – cerebrospinal fluid

PET – Photon Emission Tomography

PiB – Pittsburgh Compound B

FDDNP – 2-(1-{6-[2-[F18]fluoroethyl) (methyl) amino]-2-naphthyl}ethylidene) malononitrile

MRI FLAIR – Magnetic Resonance Imageing fluid attenuation inversion recovery

covered in Chapter 6 refers more to routine clinical practice. As AD advances, the effects of cortical changes become notable and can involve several domains – executive function, language, praxis, complex visual processing and gnosis. The emergence of neuropsychiatric symptoms, including apathy or delusions, also constitutes a clinical marker of the disease. However, even in these more advanced cases there should be evidence of an early and previous episodic memory deficit as a mandatory requirement for the diagnosis of AD.

A detailed physical examination is also an important part of the diagnostic process in dementia and this combined with other information should then result in the patient undergoing a more detailed psychiatric assessment. From a practical perspective, the GP is probably in the best position to comment on the physical health of the patient, and where this is unclear a local protocol should be developed to clarify the roles of the different healthcare professionals to make the patient's journey as smooth as possible and to avoid unnecessary duplication of work and investigations.

Following the psychiatric and medical history and physical examination a number of investigations such as kidney, liver, thyroid and other blood tests can be undertaken and additional investigation as indicated such as ECGs, chest X-rays and neuroimaging techniques (*see* below and Figure 4.1) to clarify the diagnosis and help to identify any potentially reversible case for the cognitive impairment (*see* Box 4.2 on page 61). For a more detailed examination of the physical aspects of dementia *see* Chapter 6.

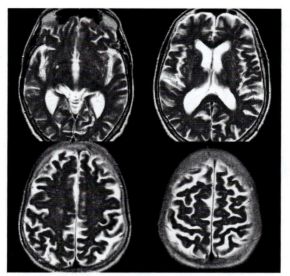

57-year-old female. MRI: Axial T2W. Generalised atrophy: widening of CSF spaces and Virchow-Robin spaces (CSF spaces surrounding vessels that perfuse the brain).

Figure 4.1 Generalised atrophy: Alzheimer's disease

Neuroimaging

There has been unprecedented growth of scientific knowledge about several types of dementias, more specifically AD. The description of distinctive and reliable biomarkers that are now available through structural brain imaging with magnetic resonance imaging (MRI), molecular neuroimaging with photon emission tomography, with the addition of cerebrospinal fluid analyses, as well as a better definition of the clinical profile of amnestic disorders that occur early in the course of the disease, make it possible to identify specifically AD with high accuracy, even in the early stages of the disease. Dubois and colleagues again proposed new criteria for the diagnosis which capture both the prodromal and the more advanced dementia stages of the disease in the same diagnostic framework.[8]

Until recently it was proposed that neuroimaging could only be used in screening programmes, and that in practice its cost means it is more useful for research purposes or for confirming the diagnosis in patients already shown to have cognitive impairment. However, with recent advances, the use of neuroimaging potentially can become a much more useful tool in both the screening and diagnostic settings of dementia.[9]

Structural neuroimaging

Structural neuroimaging is useful in the diagnostic work-up for patients with dementia, helping to exclude potentially reversible causes of dementia assess-

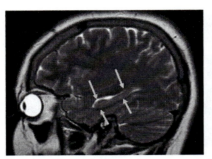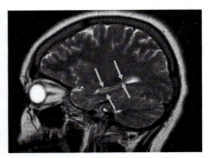

Female patient with progressive severe cognitive disorder and memory impairment. Later on she developed dementia and secondarily generalised temporal seizures. MRI: sagittal T2 weighted images showing hippocampal atrophy, on the left, and sclerosis triggering seizures, on the right.

Figure 4.2 Hippocampal atrophy

ing usually acceptable levels as normal decreasing brain volume, grey and white matter according to age.[10] Imaging techniques to study the brain include computed tomography (CT) and MRI. The latter allows obtaining detailed structural imaging analyses of the brain as an almost routine test in present clinical practice. More advanced techniques include 3-dimensional MR acquisitions, Isovoxel-based morphometry (IVBM) and tractography.

Magnetic resonance in AD has shown that entorhinal cortex volumetry and also hippocampal volumetry can discriminate between those with mild cognitive deficits and healthy controls.[11] Longitudinal studies of AD have shown that general brain atrophy in terms of total brain volume loss determined by serial MRI is in the range of 1–2.8% per year for AD, much larger than the rate of 0.05–0.41% per year for elderly controls[11] (*see* Figure 4.2).

Patients with AD also had accelerated rates of hippocampal atrophy[12,13] compared with controls, as well as focal areas of cortical atrophy, such as the precuneus,[9] on the medial aspect of the cerebral hemispheres and inferior parietal gyri both related to integrated vision of both objects and reading words.[14,15] In this regard, one of the most remarkable research works in a clinically well-known group of patients is the one encompassed by The Nuns' study,[12] carried out in the US on a group of Roman Catholic nuns living in a convent who gave consent to be clinically examined yearly, also donating their brains after natural death. Post-mortem MR and subsequent morphometric pathology exams showed strong evidence of a recognisable degree of hippocampal atrophy in those who developed dementia, an accelerated degree of atrophy in those who developed minor or moderate memory loss and an acceptable slow decline in volume of those clinically normal.[12] Common clinical MR protocols and tools for clinical research with MR using techniques such as IVBM, combining detailed volume acquisitions with adequate computer programs, are now becoming more common within the clinical domain. Similar MR procedures, based on detection of paths of diffusion of normal water molecules, also allow visualising with MR of the neural tracts assessing bundles of axons, neural pathways and physiologically active networks of neurons that may also deteriorate earlier in those patients with AD and other types of dementia. Thus MRI could be used alongside clinical assessment to detect early AD.[16] However, MRI is an expensive procedure and it is not readily available, especially for large-scale screening of community-based patients.

A recent CT scan study examined medial temporal lobe atrophy in 10 patients with mild cognitive impairment, 42 patients with AD and 29 non-demented controls. When the specificity was fixed at 95%, the sensitivity for AD was found to be 93% and for mild cognitive impairment 80%.[17]

Functional imaging

Magnetic resonance spectroscopy (MRS) has also been suggested as a useful technique for the early detection of AD. MRS is an imaging technique that can determine the amount of cerebral metabolites in the living brain, including N-acetylaspartate (NAA), choline-containing compounds (Cho), creatine-phosphocreatine (Cr), and myoinositol (MI). NAA is considered to be a neurone marker and has been extensively studied in AD, and reductions in its concentration have been found in the brains of patients with AD. MI is considered to be a tentative glial marker and to represent gliosis severity in AD.[18] It has been suggested that the severity of AD can be monitored by the relative reduction of NAA/Cr concentration ratio in the medial temporal lobe. MRS findings in other dementias have been compared with AD. On the basis of MI elevation being larger in frontotemporal dementia compared with AD, 92% of patients with frontotemporal dementia were correctly differentiated from AD (clinical differentiation). Small studies of MRS comparing AD with vascular dementia have suggested regional differences in disease distribution, with more involvement of the frontal lobe in vascular dementia and the parietal lobe in AD. It has also been found that patients with vascular dementia had lower NAA/Cr and NAA/Cho ratios in the subcortical white matter compared with patients with AD. These findings need confirmation in larger studies. In addition, MRS is not practical in clinical practice due to limited availability and poor spatial resolution, although this drawback has been significantly improved by implementing techniques of multivoxel spectroscopy of the whole brain.[19,20]

Other studies have suggested that photon emission tomography (PET) scans might be helpful. Recent findings suggest that in patients with AD, changes in the posterior cingulate, temporoparietal and prefrontal association cortex correlated with dementia severity. In patients with mild to moderate AD, the sensitivity and specificity were 93%. This fell to 84% sensitivity and 93% specificity for patients with MMSE scores ≥ 24.[21]

Another technique that has been investigated involves examining activated microglia. These have a key role in the brain's immune response to neuronal degeneration. This is associated with an increased expression of receptors known as peripheral benzodiazepine binding sites. Using PET techniques (carbon-11-labelled R-PK11195), binding properties have been shown not to change with age, but there is significantly increased binding in patients with mild AD, particularly in the entorhinal, temporoparietal and cingulate cortex.[18]

In addition, distinguishing dementia of Lewy body (DLB) from a more common type such as AD, can be very challenging. The presence of Alzheimer's pathology modifies the clinical picture of DLB. Applying the clinical diagnostic criteria for DLB at clinical presentation might fail to identify up to 50% of DLB cases. A recent study by Walker and colleagues in Essex, UK, tried to determine whether functional imaging of the nigrostriatal pathways could improve the accuracy of diagnosis compared with diagnosis by means of clinical criteria alone.[22] A single photon emission computed tomography (SPECT) scan was carried out with dopaminergic presynaptic ligand Ioflupane (FP-CIT) on a group of patients with a clinical diagnosis of DLB or other dementia. The sensitivity of the FP-CIT scan for the diagnosis of DLB increased to 88% with a specificity of 100%, compared with the sensitivity of an initial clinical diagnosis of 75% and specificity of 42%. FP-CIT SPECT scans substantially enhanced the accuracy of diagnosis of DLB in comparison with clinical criteria alone.

Biochemical tests

A number of neurological conditions clinically similar to AD are caused by transmissible agents. These include kuru, Creutzfeldt–Jakob disease (CJD) and Gerstmann–Straussler syndrome. These diseases are due to prions which, until relatively recently, were unknown infectious agents. Prions have a long incubation period with none of the inflammatory responses seen with viral infections. This raises the possibility that AD might also be caused by a transmissible agent, but evidence remains unconvincing. However, the only biochemical test that has become established in clinical practice is the measurement of the 14-3-3 proteins in cerebrospinal fluid to help diagnose sporadic cases of Creutzfeldt–Jakob disease.

Diagnostic schedules

AD, one of the common causes of dementia, can be diagnosed with high sensitivity (85%) using standardised criteria.[23] A number of diagnostic schedules are also frequently used in clinical practice including *DSM-IV* and *ICD-10* and these are discussed more fully in Chapter 3.

Box 4.2   Some causes of reversible dementia

Intra-cranial	Subdural haematoma
	Tumour
	Abscess
Central nervous system infection	Syphilis
	Tuberculosis
	Fungal infections
Endocrine	Hyper/hypothyroidism
	Hyper/hypoparathyroidism
	Hyper/hypoadrenalism
Collagen diseases	Systemic lupus erythematosus
	Temporal arteritis
Metabolic	Liver disease
	Renal disease
	Wilson's disease
	Pernicious anaemia
	Folate deficiency
Toxic	Alcohol
	Heavy metals, e.g. aluminium
Psychiatric	Depression/mania
	Schizophrenia
	Conversion disorder
	Ganser syndrome
Miscellaneous	Communicating hydrocephalus
	Epilepsy
	Parkinson's disease
	Remote effect of various cancers
	Cardiac insufficiency
	Respiratory insufficiency

SCREENING TESTS

Tests for cognitive impairment

One of the most widely used cognitive tests is the Mini-Mental State Examination (MMSE).[24] It has a high sensitivity and specificity (87%) for dementia in older people with memory impairment. It is a short cognitive test that takes 10 minutes or less to administer, it is not stressful for patients and can easily be incorporated into clinical practice with a minimal amount of training. It is a screening instrument and should not be used as a diagnostic test. Patients who have evidence of cognitive impairment need to be further evaluated, partly to establish the diagnosis of dementia and then to clarify the specific cause of the dementia.

The clock-drawing test is also clinically useful, takes only a few minutes to perform and has a sensitivity and specificity of 85% for dementia with good inter-rater reliability.[25] It taps into a wide range of cognitive abilities and is also able to detect deterioration, but cannot distinguish between the different causes of dementia. However, it is useful when language is a barrier to cognitive testing, but caution needs to be exercised when used in patients with low educational achievement.

The six-item Cognitive Impairment Test (6CIT) is an improvement on the MMSE as it is quicker to administer and outperforms it in milder dementia.[26] It should therefore prove to be a better screening tool than the MMSE for identifying milder cases of dementia that the MMSE would miss, but further work is needed to establish this.

The early detection of dementia might also be aided by a screening test that could be administered by the family. The Symptoms of Dementia Screener (SDS) is an 11-item questionnaire, designed for use by lay persons to screen for dementia, and can also be administered over the telephone.[27] A score of 5 or more is associated with a sensitivity of 90.2% and a specificity of 84.6% for dementia in community-based samples of patients with cognitive impairment.

Tests for Alzheimer's disease

In an attempt to improve the usefulness of the MMSE one retrospective pragmatic study set in a district general old age psychiatric service investigated whether the spread of scores on the seven sub-sections of the MMSE, rather than the total score could be used to classify dementia into Alzheimer's dementia and non-Alzheimer's dementia.

Case notes of those patients with cognitive decline were identified from discharge records and also by contacting the community psychiatric nurses. MMSE scores in each of the seven sub-sections (orientation, registration, attention, recall, language, three-stage command, pentagon construction), total scores and the clinical diagnosis made by the consultant were recorded. There were a total of 45 cases with dementia, 14 AD and 31 non-AD. The results showed that it was not possible to classify dementia into AD and non-AD based on the spread of scores on the seven sub-sections of the MMSE (Sood, 2003, unpublished).

The Cambridge Cognitive Examination (CAMCOG), a screening instrument, was evaluated in a data set comprising healthy subjects, subjects with incident AD and subjects with prevalent AD to investigate its ability to detect early AD.[28] The authors concluded that for the early detection of AD it was best to use the memory and non-memory scores of the test separately instead of the total score, since it was found that a low memory score in the context of a relatively good general cognition predicted early stages of AD. However, whilst this study confirmed the clinical experience that memory problems arise early in AD, it did not investigate whether the CAMCOG instrument could be used to distinguish AD from other dementias. Neither did the study establish whether the instrument could pick out AD from patients presenting to clinical practice with cognitive problems.

More recently, two subtests (paired associate learning and delayed matching) of the Cambridge Neuropsychological Test Automated Battery (CANTAB) identified all cases of early AD that subsequently met diagnostic criteria for AD.[29]

Semenza *et al.*[30] also compared the efficiency of three instruments at distinguishing subjects with AD from healthy controls. Two tests requiring proper name retrieval were prepared and compared against the MMSE[23] and the Modified MMSE (3MS).[31] It was found that the MMSE had a ceiling effect and was not able to detect milder cases of AD from the control group. The 3MS was more sensitive than the MMSE due to its 'verbal fluency sub-test' and the proper name retrieval test was more sensitive still.

Other studies did attempt to distinguish AD from other types of dementia. Mathuranath *et al.*[32] validated a simple bedside test battery (Addenbrooke's Cognitive Examination, ACE), designed to detect mild dementia and differentiate AD from frontotemporal dementia. The ACE is a 100-point test battery, assessing six cognitive areas – orientation, attention, memory, verbal fluency, language and visuospatial ability – and takes 15–20 minutes to administer. Patients with dementia were compared with a control group. It was found that the ACE had a higher sensitivity than the MMSE for the early detection of dementia and it could differentiate AD from frontotemporal dementia in mildly demented patients. Some of these tests are summarised in Table 4.2.

Other psychometric tests

Computerised adaptation of the Hayling task

The Hayling task measures the ability to inhibit semantically constrained responses. Patients with AD show a severe deficit in both error rates and response time on the Hayling task. A recent study by Bellinger and Belleville aimed to measure semantic inhibitory capacities in patients with a diagnosis of AD or mild cognitive impairment (MCI).[33] Results indicated that semantic inhibition of a prepotent response is impaired in participants with MCI and may have predictive value regarding future decline, supporting its prognostic role in the early identification of dementia.

The investigators relied on a computerised adaptation of the Hayling task, designed to diminish the likelihood of using alternative non-inhibitory

Table 4.2 Pencil and paper tests for detecting dementia

	MMSE	6CIT	SDS	CAMCOG	CANTAB	ACE
Low cost	+	+	+	+/–	+/–	+/–
Ease of use	+	+	+	+/–	+/–	+/–
Portable	+	+	+	+	+/–	+
Low risk	+	+	+	+	+	+
Detection of dementia	+/–	+	+	+	+	+
Detection of type of dementia	–	–	–	–	–	+/–
Established reliability	+/–	+	+	+	+	+
Useful in mild dementia	–	+	+/–	+	+	+
Useful in pre-clinical dementia	–	–	–	–	–	–

MMSE, Mini Mental State Examination test; 6CIT, 6-item Cognitive Impairment Test; SDS, Symptoms of Dementia Screener; CAMCOG, Cambridge Cognitive Examination; CANTAB, Cambridge Neuropsychological Test Automated Battery; ACE, Addenbrooke's Cognitive Examination.

strategies. Participants with both AD and MCI showed impaired performance on the inhibition condition. Participants with AD showed both poorer score and an increased number of errors, whereas participants with MCI obtained lower score. There was also an effect of normal ageing in the inhibition condition when considering reaction time only.

In participants with MCI and AD, there was a significant correlation between lexico-semantic capacities and performance on the automatic condition. Follow-up analysis revealed that participants with MCI who experienced a subsequent significant cognitive decline had impaired performance in the inhibition condition at the time of the experiment, while participants with MCI who remained stable did not.

Critical Flicker Fusion Threshold (CFFT)

Critical Flicker Fusion Threshold (CFFT) is a well-established neurophysiological technique that has been extensively studied in young and older healthy volunteers. The neurophysiological basis of flicker perception is well described.[34] Flickering light directly influences cortical activity (measured by electroencephalogram, EEG), and although flickering light is able to initiate neuronal activity in various parts of the visual system (from retina to cortex), the temporal resolution of CFFT appears to be determined principally by the occipital cortex. Above a particular frequency, flickering light does not appear to flicker and the point at which this occurs is the CFFT and is a measure of the information-processing capacity of the central nervous system. In the ascending mode, the frequency of flicker is gradually increased until the flickering lights appear to stop flickering – this is the ascending threshold. In the descending mode, the frequency of flicker is gradually decreased until the lights appear to start flickering – this is the descending threshold. The CFFT is the average of the ascending and descending thresholds.

CFFT has been examined in a large community sample of healthy older people (n = 644) and scores were normally distributed. Descending thresholds were significantly higher than ascending thresholds, confirming findings from studies in younger subjects. In addition, there were no significant correlations between CFFT, ascending and descending thresholds and age. However, although not significant, there was a negative correlation between age and descending thresholds. The lack of a correlation between CFFT, ascending and descending thresholds and age is important since if CFFT were correlated with age, this measure would probably be unable to distinguish change in cognitive function due to age or the disease process in a longitudinal context, e.g. as a screening instrument. In a further study, CFFT and ascending and descending thresholds were examined in patients with AD and healthy controls. CFFT and descending thresholds were significantly lower in patients with AD compared with healthy controls, whereas ascending thresholds were not significantly different in the two groups. In addition, in the patient group, ascending thresholds were also significantly higher than descending thresholds and this latter finding is a reversal of the situation seen in healthy older subjects and this might be a characteristic feature of AD. In a series of further studies in patients with AD, CFFT has also been shown to have a high test–retest reliability, high inter-rater reliability and to be a valid measure in patients with AD. These studies have been described elsewhere in more detail.[35] CFFT is quick and easy to administer as well as being cheap and portable. It requires relatively little training and has high validity and reliability in patients with AD, and would be suitable to evaluate further as a screening test.

Choice Reaction Time (CRT)

Choice Reaction Time (CRT) is a widely used measure with an extensive body of literature. Hindmarch and Wattis[36] have suggested that CRT is an indicator of sensori-motor performance, a common feature of many 'everyday' activities. It has also been proposed as a measure of the efficiency of attentional and response mechanisms in the information-processing chain, without the need for extensive cognitive processing.[35] In this test, subjects are required to respond to a critical stimulus, and the time taken to do this is recorded. However, because the subject is presented with a number of identical stimuli, this also provides a measure of attentional monitoring abilities. A number of studies have demonstrated significant reductions in reaction times in patients with AD compared with controls,[37,38] and because of its ease of use it should be investigated further as a screening test. These tests are summarised in Table 4.3.

Table 4.3 Clinical assessment and psychometric tests for detecting dementia

	Clinical diagnosis	CFFT	CRT	Computerised adaptation of the Hayling task
Low cost	–	+	+	+
Ease of use	–	+/–	+/–	+/–
Portable	+	+	+	+
Low risk	+	+	+	+
Detection of dementia	+	+	?	+
Detection of type of dementia	+	+/–	?	–
Established reliability	+	+	?	–
Useful in mild dementia	+/–	+	?	+
Useful in pre-clinical dementia	–	+/–	?	+/–

CFFT, Critical Flicker Fusion Threshold; CRT, Choice Reaction Time.

Electroencephalogram (EEG)

The EEG is a potentially useful measure in patients with AD, and slowing of alpha frequency and increased theta and delta activity are observed as the condition progresses. Differences tend to be greater during rest with eyes open and in one recent study the test was able to correctly classify 77% of patients with mild AD.[39]

Magnetoencepahlography (MEG)

Magnetoencepahlography (MEG), like other magnetic resonance techniques, is based on Faraday's Law of Induction, which states that every magnetic field generates an electrical impulse and vice versa. The MEG unit is a special magnet, shaped like a small helmet, that is placed on the head like a hat. It also has special marking points, making it useful to fuse the exquisite sensitivity of MEG with the special resolution afforded by MRI. Its advantage is mainly functional, studying cortex activation after stimuli that may be as simple as naming the letters of the alphabet, reading a complex text or measuring extension of cortical activation on more complex cognitive tasks, short-term memory, word association and spatial resolution memory. Unfortunately, applicability as an extensive diagnostic test, even in high-risk patients, does not appear as a realistic possibility at the moment due to its cost, although it can be used in selected borderline patients or as a research tool.

Event-related potentials (ERPs)

Event-related potentials (ERPs) are changes in brain electrical activity, as recorded by scalp electrodes, in response to external stimulation of one of the many sensory tracts in the brain. Hence auditory ERPs can be recorded over the auditory brain cortex in response to the subject listening to an auditory stimulus. The subject is presented with two slightly different stimuli, one frequently and the other rarely (the 'oddball'). Signal averaging detects the potential generated in response to the 'oddball' (called the 'oddball ERP'). ERPs are plots of microvolts against time and have the appearance of several waves. Each component wave is named according to whether it is a negative (N) or positive (P) deflection. ERPs have been studied in a variety of conditions.

In a case control study,[40] abnormalities in the oddball ERP have been observed in those at increased risk for developing AD (i.e. those who have family history of AD or who carry the apolipoprotien E ε4 allele) (*see* Chapter 3). These changes were observed in the absence of neuropsychological deficits. It therefore seems that AD has a pre-clinical stage and early detection should theoretically be possible. There is some evidence that in familial AD, episodic memory problems predate the onset of AD with clear signs of progression.[41] In this study, AD was diagnosed according to National Institute of Neurological and Communicative Disorders and Stroke, AD and Related Disorders Association criteria. This study showed that more subtle cognitive changes predate other more obvious cognitive changes. Some of the neuroimaging and electrophysiological techniques are summarised in Table 4.4.

Table 4.4 Neuroimaging and electrophysiological tests for detecting dementia

	MRI	CT	MRS	PET	EEG	ERP
Low cost	–	–	–	–	–	–
Ease of use	–	–	–	–	–	–
Portable	–	–	–	–	–	–
Low risk	+/–	+/–	+/–	+/–	+	+
Detection of dementia	+	+	+	+	+/–	+
Detection of type of dementia	+	+	+	+	+/–	+/–
Established reliability	+	+	+	+	+	+
Useful in mild dementia	+	+	+/– research centres	+/– research centres	+/– research centres	+/– research centres
Useful in pre-clinical dementia	+/–	–	?	?	?	?

MRI, Magnetic Resonance Imageing; CT, Computerised Tomography; MRS, Magnetic Resonance Spectroscopy; PET, Photon Emission Tomography; EEG, Electroencephalogram; ERP, Event Related Potential.

Biochemical tests

The idea that biomarkers appear during the pre-clinical phase of dementia, and more specific AD, has led to the expansion of research studies into this field. It has become possible now to detect biomarkers such as soluble Aβ 42 before the deposits of amyloid plaques and neurofibrillary tangles appear. This occurs prior to the deterioration of cognitive functioning and the decline of the instrumental activity of daily living. These methods increase the hope for early diagnosis, differential diagnosis and intervention in dementia and AD.[42] Combining CSF-tau and CSF-Aβ 1-42 allows differential diagnosis between AD and normal ageing as well as other neurological disorders, such as depression, therefore allowing early diagnosis of AD. Adding phospho-tau181p quantification allows improved differential diagnosis between AD and non-AD dementia. Galasko, Kanai and Hulstaert and their respective colleagues have shown just this in studies.[43]

Acetylcholine, a neurotransmitter involved in memory mechanisms, is found predominantly in the cerebral cortex, caudate nucleus and parts of the limbic system. The presence of this neurotransmitter can be indirectly assessed by the presence of either the synthetic enzyme choline acetyltransferase (CAT), or the metabolic enzyme, acetylcholinesterase (AChE). By measuring these enzymes, it has been shown that there is an age-dependent reduction in CAT and that CAT concentrations are also decreased in patients with AD, but these findings have not led to any clinically useful test.

A reliable serum marker for early AD and other causes of dementia would be helpful and a number of candidate markers have been suggested. Recently, Lewczuk and colleagues measured concentrations of Aβ peptides 1-42 and 1-40, and their ratio in plasma of patients carefully categorised clinically and neurochemically as having AD or other dementias.[44] They used a newly commercially available multiplexing assay, characterised by reasonable laboratory performance. Patients with AD or mild cognitive impairment of AD type (MCI-AD) whose clinical diagnosis was supported with CSF biomarkers ($n = 193$) had significantly lower Aβ 1-42 plasma concentrations ($p < 0.007$), and Aβ 1-42/1-40 ratios ($p < 0.003$) compared with patients with other dementias and MCI of other types ($n = 64$). No significant differences between patients with MCI of AD type and patients with early AD were observed, or between MCI of other types and patients with early dementia of other types. Their findings reconfirmed the hypothesis that alterations of biomarker concentrations occur early in a preclinical AD stage and that these alterations are also reflected in plasma.

Levels of α1-antichymotrypsin (a protein which is released from the liver during acute inflammatory states) have been measured in the serum and cerebrospinal fluid of patients with AD and vascular dementia.[45] However, the study was relatively small, involving only 74 subjects. There was much overlap in the raised cerebrospinal fluid levels between the three groups (AD patients, vascular dementia patients and the control group). However, raised levels above 0.75% of the total CSF protein were highly specific for AD, with a specificity of 100%, but a sensitivity of only 25.6%. Larger studies would be useful to confirm this finding.

Tau protein and β-amyloid in the CSF have also been suggested as possible markers for the early detection of AD, and Blennow *et al.*[46] concluded that they are particularly useful for discriminating between age-associated memory impairment, depression and secondary causes of dementia. However, this is not a universal view and Green[47] has suggested that these markers do not have sufficient sensitivity and specificity for clinical use.

Another possibility is the AD-associated neuronal thread protein gene that encodes a 41 kD membrane-spanning phosphoprotein. This gene is over-expressed in AD, and this is said to begin early in the course of the disease. This protein is released or secreted by dying cells into the cerebrospinal fluid. These elevated levels can be detected and the most recent assay, termed 7cGold ,has greater than 90% specificity and sensitivity.[48]

No major technical or ethical issues were found that would hamper the procedure's ability to become routine in early and differential diagnostics of AD. Cut-off values for β-amyloid (median 500; range 300–849 pg/mL), total tau (367; 195–450 pg/mL) and phosphorylated tau (60; 40–85 pg/mL) varied considerably amongst countries, and even within every country. This observation yields a potential threat to an interpretation and balanced use in clinical practice. An automatic recommendation follows, therefore, that each laboratory has to establish normative data and that multi-centred studies should be organised to explore the reasons for any differences. Even if a CSF-based test proved to be helpful as a diagnostic test, it is unlikely to be helpful from a practical perspective for screening large numbers of people with mild or pre-clinical AD as it is time-consuming and relatively expensive and the procedure is invasive, uncomfortable, occasionally painful and potentially dangerous. At this stage it is unlikely to move beyond a potential research tool.

There has also been a long-standing interest in free radicals. These are atoms or molecules with one or more unpaired electrons and are particularly likely to arise in chemical reactions involving oxygen. When oxygen is chemically reduced, free radicals may be formed, including the superoxide and hydroxyl radicals. These interact with other molecules to produce new free radicals and thus set in motion a 'chain reaction'. Such substances are particularly toxic to biological molecules (e.g. DNA and proteins) and, to deal with them, the body uses a number of natural defences, including enzymes (e.g. superoxide dismutase) and antioxidants (e.g. vitamin E).[49] It has been suggested that free radical reactions are the cause of ageing and AD. This is said to be due to the progressive accumulation of irreversible damage caused by free radicals, but to date no clinically useful test has been developed. These are summarised in Table 4.5.

Brain biopsy

This is unlikely to ever be a viable screening test. It is an invasive technique and would raise a number of practical and ethical concerns including patient

Table 4.5 Biochemical, olfactory and biopsy tests for the detection of dementia

	Blood tests	CSF tests	Brain biopsy	Olfactory tests
Low cost	+/−	−	−	+
Ease of use	+/−	−	−	+/−
Portable	+/−	−	−	+
Low risk	+/−	−	−	+
Detection of dementia	−	+/−	+/−	+/−
Detection of type of dementia	−	+/− *	+	+/−
Established reliability	+	+	+	?
Useful in mild dementia	−	+/−	+/−	?
Useful in pre-clinical dementia	−	−	−	?

* The only established test is measurement of the protein 14-3-3 in CSF for Creutzfeldt–Jakob disease

safety, issues to do with the handling and storage of tissue samples, difficulties related to consent and problems associated with using the procedure on large numbers of people. Although the microscopic examination of such samples is often portrayed as a diagnostic 'gold standard', it is frequently difficult to distinguish between brain changes seen in healthy older people and the pathological features of early AD. Some of the changes seen in healthy older people include decreased brain weight, decreased brain volume, dendritic loss, widening of sulci and ventricles, neuritic plaques, neurofibrillary tangles and deposits of lipofuscin, aluminium, copper, iron and melanin. These changes are also the primary neuropathological features seen in AD.

During the first 50 years in healthy people, grey matter is lost at a greater rate than white matter, but during the second 50 years, white matter is lost at a greater rate. The loss in patients with AD is similar but greater, i.e. there is a quantitative rather than a qualitative difference, and for these reasons some authors have suggested that AD may simply be an exaggeration of the healthy ageing process.

Neuritic plaques, the neuropathological hallmark of AD, are extracellular aggregates, 50–200 μm in diameter, within the neuropil of the brain (that part of the grey matter between neurones consisting mainly of neuronal processes). The main constituent of amyloid is amyloid β protein, which is also known as βA4 and Aβ. Hardy and Higgins[50] have put forward the 'amyloid cascade hypothesis', in which they proposed that βA4 is directly or indirectly neurotoxic and that this leads to the development of neuritic plaques and neurofibrillary tangles, with subsequent neuronal cell death. βA4 is derived from another larger protein called amyloid precursor protein (APP), which has several different isoforms and is a trans-membrane protein. However, the exact function of APP is unknown, although it may be important in maintaining the integrity of synapses. Interestingly, it has been known for some time that patients with Down's syndrome (trisomy 21) who live into their 50s also develop neuropathological features of AD, and the gene for APP has been localised on chromosome 21. Neurofibrillary tangles are lesions within the cytoplasm of the perikaryon of medium and large pyramidal cells of the neo- and paleocortex. They occur less frequently in the subcortical nuclei. Under the electron microscope they can be seen as paired helical filaments, but precisely how they impair cortical function is not known.

Although the pathological features of AD are well known, it is unlikely that brain biopsy will be widely used because of practical and safety considerations, and also because of the considerable overlap with the changes seen in healthy ageing.

Olfactory tests

Deficits in both odour detection and odour identification occur in patients with AD.[49] Odour identification deficits arise earlier than odour detection problems, presumably because the latter requires less cognitive functioning than the former. The utility of olfactory testing for differential diagnosis of dementia is limited. However, against healthy controls, odour identification tests have a correct classification rate (sensitivity) of 83–100%.[51] Perhaps such tests, which only take 5–10 minutes to administer, should be seriously considered for use as part of the diagnostic work-up in AD and should be investigated more fully.

The usefulness of olfactory mucosal biopsy has been proposed for the early diagnosis of AD. However, there is controversy as to the usefulness of such biopsy, since no pathognomic changes to date have been found.[52]

Olfactory detection decreases with increasing age, but this is significantly greater in patients with AD.[53]

Genetic tests

This is a rapidly developing area and will undoubtedly be important for increasing our understanding of the aetiology of AD. It is less helpful in terms of diagnosis as a positive test does not predict when an individual patient will develop the condition. However, if an increased risk is identified, patients could be carefully monitored, perhaps every six months, and treatment started as soon as symptoms develop. It could also be useful in pre-clinical treatment using an enriched sample. Such treatment would be unsuitable for the general population but reserved for those at high risk based on their genetic profile. In the near future it is also likely to become increasingly important in the field of pharmacogenetics, where a particular genetic profile might guide which drug was prescribed. For more information on the genetics of AD *see* Chapter 3.

CONCLUSIONS

Dementia is a global phenomenon with extensive healthcare, societal and economical implications. Alzheimer' disease is the fourth leading cause of death, after heart disease, cancer and stroke. Early diagnosis of dementia has clear advantages for any patient, their carers and also health professionals with regards to planning early and successful, considerate treatments. Even though there is currently considerable overlap between screening and diagnostic testing, continuous advances in these fields improve the validity and reduce the uncertainty, which can be a diagnostic minefield. Pencil and paper tests such as the mini mental state examination test should be used for screening, and tests such as critical flicker fusion may have an additional advantage in very early detection. Other measures such as neuroimaging and biochemical tests are more suited to clarifying diagnosis and might be used more frequently in the clinical setting after screening and for ongoing research.

Key points

➤ Early diagnosis of dementia is important to help professionals, patients and their families plan for the future and increase the chances that treatments will be effective.

➤ If detected early, some dementias can be reversed, such as normal pressure hydrocephalus, some can be stabilised thus preventing further progression, including some vascular dementias, and some can have their progression slowed, such as Alzheimer's disease.

➤ Simple screening tests that identify cognitive impairment combined with further investigations are currently the best strategy for diagnosing dementia and the different sub-types.

➤ No confirmed diagnostic test for Alzheimer's disease has yet been identified; however, candidate tests, including blood tests and CSF parameters, are being developed.

REFERENCES

1 Stewart R. Cardiovascular factors in Alzheimers disease. *Journal of Neurology, Neurosurgery and Psychiatry*. 1998; **65**: 143–7.

2 Bullock R. New drugs for Alzheimer's disease and other dementias. *British Journal of Psychiatry*. 2002; **180**: 131–9.

3 Forlenza OV, Dinis BS, Nunes PV, *et al.* Diagnostic transitions in mild cognitive impairment subtypes. *International Psychogeriatrics*. 2009; **21**(6): 1088–95.

4 Thambisetty M, Simmonds A, Velayudhan L, *et al.* Association of plasma clusterin concentration with severity, pathology and progression in Alzheimer's disease. *Archives of General Psychiatry*. 2010; **67**(7): 739–48.

5   Greenhalgh T. *How to Read a Paper: the basics of evidence based medicine*. 4th ed. Oxford: Wiley-Blackwell/BMJ Books; 2010. pp. 98–112.

6   Simic G, Stanic G, Mladinov M. Does Alzheimer's disease begin in the brainstem? *Neuropathology Applied Neurobiology*. 2009; 35(6): 532–54.

7   Dubois B, Feldman H, Scheltens, P. A new concept and new criteria for Alzheimer's disease. *European Neurological Disease*. 2007; Issue II.

8   Dubois B, Picard G, Sarazin M. Early detection of Alzheimer's disease: new diagnostic criteria. *Dialogues Clin Neurosci*. 2009; 11(2): 135–9.

9   Karas G, Scheltens P, Rombouts S, *et al*. Precuneus atrophy in early-onset Alzheimer's disease: a morphometric structural MRI study. *Neuroradiology*. 2007; 49: 967–76.

10 Courchesne E, Chisum H, Townsend J, *et al*. Normal brain development and ageing: quantitative analysis at in vivo MR imaging in healthy volunteers. *Radiology*. 2000; **216**: 672–82.

11 Hsu YY, Du AT, Wiener MW, *et al*. Magnetic resonance imaging and magnetic resonance spectroscopy in dementias. *Journal of Geriatric Psychiatry and Neurology*. 2001; 14(3): 145–66.

12 Gosche KM, Mortimer JA, Smith CD, *et al*. Hippocampal volume as an index of Alzheimer neuropathology: findings from the Nun Study. *Neurology*. 2002; **58**: 1476–82.

13 Gosche KM, Mortimer JA, Smith CD, *et al*. An automated technique for measuring hippocampal volumes from MR imaging studies. *AJNR Am J Neuroradiol*. 2001; **22**: 1686–9.

14 McKeefry DJ, Gouws A, Burton MP, *et al*. The non-invasive dissection of the human visual cortex using fMRI and TMS to study the organisation of vision in the brain. *Neuroscientist*. 2009; **15**: 489–506.

15 Shafriz KM, Gore JC, Marois R: The role of the parietal cortex in visual feature binding. *PNAS*. 2002; 99(16): 10917–22.

16 Chetelat G, Baron JC. Early diagnosis of Alzheimer's disease; contribution of structural imaging. *Neuroimage*. 2003; 18(2): 525–41.

17 Frisoni GB, Rossi R, Beltramello A. The radial width of the temporal horn in mild cognitive impairment. *Neuroimaging*. 2002; 12(4): 351.

18 Cagnin A, Brooks DJ, Kennedy AM, *et al*. In-vivo measurement of activated microglia in dementia. *Lancet*. 2001; **358**: 766.

19 Ackl N, Ising M, Schreiber YA, *et al*. Hippocampal metabolic abnormalities in mild cognitive impairment and Alzheimer's disease. *Neurosci Lett*. 2005; 384(1–2): 23–8.

20 Kizu O, Yamada K, Ito H, *et al*. Posterior cingulate metabolic changes in frontotemporal lobar degeneration detected by magnetic resonance spectroscopy. *Neuroradiology*. 2004; 46(4): 277–81.

21 Herol K, Salmon E, Perani D, *et al*. Discrimination between Alzheimer dementia and controls by automated analysis of multicenter FDG PET. *Neuroimage*. 2002; 17(1): 302–316.

22 Wallker Z, Jaros E, Walker RWH, *et al*. Dementia with Lewy bodies: a comparison of clinical diagnosis, FP-CIT single photon emission computed tomography imaging and autopsy. *J Neurol Neurosurg Psychiatry*. 2007; **78**: 1176–81.

23 Villareal DT, Morris JC. The diagnosis of Alzheimer's disease. *Journal of Alzheimer's Disease*. 1999; **1**: 249–63.

24 Folstein MF, Folstien S E, McHugh PR. 'Mini-mental State': A practical method for

grading the cognitive state of patients for the clinician. *Journal of Psychiatric Research*. 1975; **12**: 189–98.

25 Shulman KI. Clock drawing: is it the ideal cognitive screening test? *International Journal of Geriatric Psychiatry*. 2000; **15**: 548–61.

26 Brooke P, Bullock R. Validation of a 6 item cognitive impairment test with a view to primary care usage. *International Journal of Geriatric Psychiatry*. 1999; **14**: 936–40.

27 Mundt JC, Freed D M, Greist JH. Lay person-based screening for early detection of Alzheimer's disease: development and validation of an instrument. *Journal of Gerontology: Psychological Sciences*. 2000; **55(B)**(3): 163–70.

28 Schmand B, Walstra G, Lindeboom J, *et al*. Early detection of Alzheimer's disease using the Cambridge Cognitive Examination (CAMCOG). *Psychological Medicine*. 2000; **30**: 619–27.

29 Fowler KS, Saling MM, Conway EL, *et al*. Paired associate performance in the early detection of DAT. *Journal of International Neuropsychology and Sociology*. 2002; **8**: 58–71.

30 Semenza C, Borgo F, Mondini S, *et al*. Proper names in the early stages of Alzheimer's disease. *Brain Cognition*. 2000; **43**: 384–7.

31 Teng E L, Chui HC. The modified Mini-Mental State (3MS) examination. *Journal of Clinical Psychiatry*. 1987; **48**: 314–18.

32 Mathuranath PD, Nestor PJ, Berrios GE, *et al*. A brief cognitive test battery to differentiate Alzheimer's disease and frontotemporal dementia. *Neurology*. 2000; **55**: 1613–20.

33 Belanger S, Belleville S. Semantic inhibition impairment in mild cognitive impairment: a distinctive feature of upcoming cognitive decline? *Neuropsychology*. 2009; **23**(5): 592–606.

34 Curran S, Wattis JPW. Critical flicker fusion threshold: a potentially useful measure for the early detection of Alzheimer's disease. *Human Psychopharmacology*. 2000; **15**: 103–12.

35 Sherwood N. Effects of nicotine on human psychomotor performance. *Human Psychopharmacology, Clinical and Experimental*. 1993; **8**(3): 155–84.

36 Hindmarch I, Wattis JP. Measuring the effects of psychotropic drugs. In: Wattis JP, Hindmarch I. *Psychological Assessment of the Elderly*. Edinburgh: Churchill Livingstone; 1988. pp. 180–97.

37 Simpson PM, Surmon DJ, Wesnes KA, *et al*. The cognitive Drug Research Computerised Assessment System for demented patients: a validation study. *International Journal of Geriatric Psychiatry*. 1991; **6**: 95–102.

38 Miller E, Morris R. *The Psychology of Dementia*. Chichester: John Wiley & Sons; 1993.

39 Stevens A, Kircher T, Nickola M, *et al*. Dynamic regulation of EEG power and coherence is lost early and globally in probable DAT. *European Archives of Psychiatry and Clinical Neuroscience*. 2001; **251**: 199–204.

40 Green J, Levey AI. Event-related potential changes in groups at increased risk for Alzheimer's disease. *Archives of Neurology*. 1999; **56**(11): 1398–1403.

41 Fox NC, Warrington EK, Seiffer AL, *et al*. Presymptomatic cognitive deficits in individuals at risk of familial Alzheimer's disease. *Brain*. 1998; **121**: 1631–9.

42 Vanderberghe R. The new face of and old age disease: early diagnosis and treatment of Alzheimer's disease. Presented orally at: 'Therapy day', 2002 Oct. 5, Leuven, Belgium.

43 Galasko D, *et al.*; Kanai M, *et al.*; Hulstaert F, *et al. Arch Neurol.* 1998; **55**: 937–45. *Ann Neurol.* 1998; **44**: 17–26. *Neurol.* 1999; **52**: 1555–62.

44 Lewczuk P, Kornhuber J, Vanmechelen E. Amyloid beta peptides in plasma in early diagnosis of Alzheimer's disease: A multicenter study with multiplexing. *Exp Neurol.* 2010; **223**(2): 366–70.

45 Licastro F, Parnetti L, Morini M C, *et al.* Acute phase reactant α1-antichymotrypsin is increased in cerebrospinal fluid and serum of patients with probable Alzheimer's disease. *Alzheimer Disease and Associated Disorders.* 1995; **9**(2): 112–18.

46 Blennow K, Vanmechelen E, Hampel H. CSF total tau, Abeta42 and phosphorylated tau protein as biomarkers for Alzheimer's disease. *Molecular Neurobiology.* 2001; **24**: 87–97.

47 Green A Biochemical investigations in patients with dementia. *Annals of Clinical Biochemistry.* 2002; **39**: 211–20.

48 de la Monte SM, Wands JR. The AD7c-ntp neuronal thread protein biomarker for detecting Alzheimer's disease. *Front Bioscience.* 2002; **7**: 989–96.

49 Jorm AF. *The Epidemiology of Alzheimer's Disease and Related Disorders.* London: Chapman and Hall; 1990. pp. 54–76, 77–86, 151–70.

50 Hardy JA, Higgins GA. Alzheimer's disease: the amyloid cascade hypothesis. *Science.* 1992; **256**: 184–5.

51 Morgan CD, Nordin S, Murphy C. Odour identification is an early marker for Alzheimer's disease: impact of lexical functioning and detection sensitivity. *Journal of Clinical and Experimental Neuropsychology.* 1995; **17**(5): 793–803.

52 Kishikawa M, Sakae MIM, Kawaguchi S, *et al.* Early diagnosis of Alzheimer's? *Nature.* 1994; **369**: 365–6.

53 Lange R, Donathan CL, Hughes LF. Assessing olfactory abilities with the University of Pennsylvania smell identification test; a Rasch scaling approach. *Journal of Alzheimer's Disease.* 2002; **4**: 77–91.

CHAPTER 5

The role of the clinical psychologist in the assessment, diagnosis and management of patients with dementia

Edgar Miller

INTRODUCTION

The very concept 'dementia' is psychological in that it implies, above all else, a deterioration in psychological functioning. It is this deterioration in mental functioning that is the central feature of dementia and results in the major practical problems posed by this group of disorders. For this reason, psychological factors are essential considerations in diagnosis and management for all those who deal with those who suffer from dementing illness. In this sense, the psychological aspects of dementia go much wider than the contribution made by psychologists, although there is clearly a role for the psychologist. It is the particular contribution of the clinical psychologist to the evaluation and management of those with dementia that is the focus of this chapter.

The practical contribution made by the psychologist has two major aspects. The first is that of the psychological assessment and diagnosis of dementia, often involving the use of psychometric tests. The second major contribution is to management. These two aspects will be considered separately.

ASSESSMENT AND DIAGNOSIS

Psychological assessment of the person with dementia or possible dementia can be designed to achieve three possible aims:[1]

➤ as a means of assisting in the diagnosis of dementia

> ➤ to monitor change
> ➤ to make decisions about management.

Diagnostic assessment is the best developed of these areas and the present discussion will concentrate on this aspect and then make a few comments about other aspects of assessment.

Before commenting on assessments of different kinds, it is useful to draw attention to two sets of problems which complicate the psychological assessment of those with actual or possible Alzheimer's disease or other dementing illness.[2] Firstly, those assessed tend to be older and older people are subject to sensory loss and to physical problems, such as cardiovascular disease, which might impair psychological functioning.[3] Secondly, although the picture is improving, many potentially useful psychological tests do not have norms for older age groups and this presents a limitation on the range of instruments that can be used. This is especially a problem with regard to those who are over 75 or 80 years of age, although the situation is slowly improving.

Whilst these two problems apply generally, there is a further set of difficulties that emerges when trying to assess people from different language and cultural backgrounds. This is especially the case for those immigrants born outside the UK whose first language is not English, and for these there is, as yet, no satisfactory solution. Generally speaking, those members of immigrant communities who have been raised and educated in the UK tend to perform similarly on psychometric tests to the indigenous population, but they may still score a little less well on some instruments because of cultural differences.

Diagnostic assessment

A major underlying problem with diagnostic assessment is that diagnosis is a key issue at the point at which the individual first presents to services with problems, and this is usually early in the course of the disorder. At this time, any psychological changes are likely to be small, and the key difficulty is the problem of detecting small changes in psychological functioning, especially when it is typically the case that there is no reliable information as to how the individual might have performed on psychological tests prior to the onset of the possible dementing illness.

Screening tests

A number of screening tests for dementia have been developed. These tend to be administered more by psychiatrists than by psychologists and they are mentioned for completeness. The best known of these and possibly the best validated is the Mini-Mental State Examination of Folstein *et al.,*[4] although there are a number of similar scales available. These tend to embody a series of questions incorporating such things as general knowledge questions (e.g. 'Who is the Prime Minister?') and very simple memory tasks. The MMSE emerges as having useful, if far from perfect, levels of validity,[5] and the key items in such scales that are most effective in discriminating those with dementia are questions relating to memory and orientation.

Intelligence

As already indicated, the term 'dementia' suggests a decline in psychological functioning and especially in intellectual or cognitive functions. This might suggest that intelligence tests would play a major role in the assessment of dementia. In practice, the role of intelligence (IQ) tests of the kind exemplified by the commonly used Wechsler intelligence scales is rather limited.[6] One important reason for this is technical, in that the methods used to construct intelligence scales mean that they are relatively insensitive in reflecting small changes in functioning. It is, of course, in the early stages of dementia, before deterioration has progressed very far, that diagnosis is most difficult and where the potential contribution that psychometric tests might make to diagnosis would be most useful. As dementia progresses, it becomes easier to diagnose on clinical grounds and the value of formal testing is reduced.

Another problem in the use of intelligence tests to detect dementia is that for most people being assessed there will be no accurate indication as to the pre-morbid level of intelligence, and without some indication of this it is difficult to say if any decline in IQ has occurred based on an assessment of current IQ. Various methods of determining pre-morbid IQ have been suggested but the most satisfactory so far has proved to be the National Adult Reading Test (NART). This was originally developed in 1978,[7] but has been subsequently updated. Fuller discussions of the use of the NART to estimate pre-morbid intelligence are provided elsewhere.[8,9]

The NART works on the principle that the ability to read words appears to be highly resistant to deterioration, at least in the early stages of a progressive disorder like dementia. The test contains a set of 50 words whose spellings are irregular (e.g. 'naïve' or 'juggernaut') and which the person being tested would not be able to read out loud with correct pronunciation unless they were already familiar with the words. The ability to read irregular words in this way correlates highly with IQ and so performance on this test can be used to indicate pre-morbid IQ.

Memory

Commonly, the earliest change to be noted in someone who is developing dementia is in memory. The sufferer is noted to be more forgetful than used to be the case. In line with this, tests of memory have generally proved to be the most reliable early psychological indices of dementia. There are many different memory tests and again this discussion will be confined to a small number of examples with the works cited giving access to a much wider range of tests and a much more detailed analysis of their use in this context.

One of the most commonly used memory tests is the Wechsler Memory Scale, which is now in its third major revision.[10] In brief, this consists of a number of subtests dealing with different aspects of memory (verbal vs. non-verbal, short-term vs. long-term, etc.). The fact that this is a commonly used scale means that published data on its use has become readily available and its coverage of different aspects of memory is more comprehensive than most alternative tests of memory. Its main disadvantage arises out of that comprehensiveness, in that the full scale does take a long time to administer, which might reduce its acceptability with elderly patients.

Other useful memory tests with some standardisation data for elderly people are the Recognition Memory Test[11] and the Rivermead Behavioural Memory Test.[12] The former is a recognition test where verbal stimuli (words) or non-verbal (faces) are presented and then have to be subsequently recognised. The latter is an attempt to develop a more 'ecologically valid' memory test that tries to mimic the demands of everyday life. For example, one subtest requires that the person tested remembers to carry out an action when cued to do so by a bell. Whilst the allegedly ecological relevance of the Rivermead test makes it attractive, the levels of reliability of its subscales are less than would be desirable.

As indicated above, tests of memory have proved to be the most reliable of all psychological tests in detecting dementia and, therefore, any assessment of possible dementia needs to evaluate memory. However, two cautions should be noted. Firstly, for those who have always had low IQ levels (at around an IQ of 80 or below), poor performance on tests of memory can quite commonly occur in the absence of anything that might cause a memory loss. This makes memory testing for diagnostic purposes unreliable below this IQ level. Secondly, most of those who go to their doctors complaining of memory loss do not turn out to have dementia.[13] Usually they turn out to have some functional psychiatric disorder, commonly depression, or no disorder at all is ever identified. Interestingly, where a relative (often the spouse) complains of memory loss in the partner, this is more likely to be indicative of some form of dementia in the partner.

Other specific functions

Dementia produces deterioration in all psychological functions. In consequence, evaluation of almost any aspect of functioning can be of potential value in identifying dementia. Probably of most value in examining cases of potential dementia are tests of language and visuospatial ability.[14,15]

With respect to language, Miller set out the view that the 'first changes to be noticed are usually a general poverty of vocabulary and range of expression; speech becomes circumlocutory and repetitive … dysphasic signs may also appear at some stage of the illness'.[16] Impairments in naming are common and can be readily assessed using such instruments as the Graded Naming Test.[17] The appreciation of spatial relationships similarly tends to decline and often from quite an early stage in the disease process. Benton has developed a useful instrument to assess visuospatial functioning.[18]

Test batteries and diagnostic systems

A number of more elaborate diagnostic systems for dementia have been developed and these rely on medical/psychiatric features as well as psychological measures. The two main British examples are the CAMDEX system[19] and AGE-CAT.[20] These take a considerable length of time to administer but offer high levels of diagnostic discrimination. They are often used as research tools.

Similar tools have been developed in America. One of the most prominent of these is provided by the NINCDS-ADRDA criteria.[21,22] These have similar advantages and disadvantages to the CAMDEX and AGECAT and are again most commonly used in research settings rather than routine clinical practice.

Whilst psychological assessment can make a valuable contribution to the identification or diagnosis of dementia, they, like other forms of assessment (clinical, radiological, etc.), are far from perfect for this purpose. In general terms, normal levels of performance on cognitive tests (memory, language, etc.) can almost always be taken as excluding dementia (except for initially high-performing individuals in the very earliest stages). Poor performance on such tests has value in pointing to a dementing illness but should not be regarded as diagnostic on its own. This is because there are a number of other reasons why test performance can decline. For example, there is evidence that some people who are very depressed may do badly.[2]

A second caution is that psychological assessment on its own should not be regarded as a reliable indicator of the type of dementia. Whilst some studies have shown that, for example, multi-infarct dementia does give a different pattern of performance on psychological tests from that of Alzheimer's disease, the overlap between groups is considerable, which makes the differentiation of individual cases difficult and subject to considerable error.

Finally, whilst it is the case that patients with different forms of dementia (e.g. Alzheimer-type as opposed to cerebrovascular) do tend to have slightly different patterns of performance on psychological tests, there is always considerable overlap between the different groups. This tends to make psychological assessment much more reliable as a means of identifying some form of dementing illness than it is in distinguishing the type of dementia should such be present.

MONITORING CHANGE

The measurement of ongoing change in dementia has potential importance both from the point of view of tracking change in the individual and also in the evaluation of possible pharmacological agents that may slow down or even halt the underlying pathological process. This presents considerable technical difficulties in terms of developing measures that will be sensitive to relatively small amounts of change in such functions as memory. These problems are discussed elsewhere.[1,23]

PLANNING MANAGEMENT

Again this is something that cannot be described in detail due to limitations of space – a more detailed account is provided elsewhere.[1] Such things as scales to assess 'activities of daily living' as developed by occupational therapists and the general set of techniques known as 'behavioural assessment' can be utilised in making decisions about, for example, whether individuals can be relied on to do certain things for themselves or in determining whether special intervention programmes might be useful.[24,25]

Psychological interventions

Given that the causes of dementia lie in brain pathology, psychological interventions are not going to halt or reverse the underlying pathological processes. However, there is increasing evidence that psychological or psychosocial interventions can help maintain functioning in those who suffer from dementia, so allowing them to live as fully and independently as possible.

Environmental manipulations

The impact of the organisation and arrangement of residential units on the functioning of residents with dementia has been extensively demonstrated. For example, an early study showed that arranging the chairs in a ward dayroom so that they were grouped round small tables rather than set in lines, as had been the case, improved the level of social interaction between residents.[26]

More recent work has demonstrated the impact of enhanced stimulation.[27] This might be expected to be helpful in that many residential units provide little stimulation and an unchanging, monotonous environment. In one investigation, music appeared to be especially effective in increasing social interaction and enhancing the recall of personal information.[28]

As counter to the above, it has also been argued that overstimulation may be unhelpful for people with dementia and lead to confusion.[29] Many care settings can be rather noisy with too much going on around the person. The best practice would appear to involve the person in a level of activity that is appropriately stimulating and enjoyable without going to the extremes of monotony and understimulation, on the one hand, or a stimulus overload on the other.

Special forms of intervention

A number of special forms of intervention for people with dementia have been devised. The first and possibly best known of these is reality orientation (RO).[27] In brief, this was based on the notion that a key problem in those with dementia is that they become disoriented for place, time and person. RO is then delivered in two ways. Firstly, a 24-hour RO involves changes in the environment involving such things as use of notices and clear signposting of key locations around the ward. Staff in interaction with patients also stress information relating to orientation (e.g. by being assiduous in referring to an individual by name and mentioning the time when relevant). Secondly, there are special RO sessions in which small groups of residents meet with staff members on a regular basis for about 40 minutes at a time. Originally, these involved stressing information relating to orientation, i.e. starting by going round each member of the group by name, discussing things going on at the time of year (e.g. the presence of spring flowers) and so on. In some manifestations of RO, these activities have been greatly extended to include a wider range of things (e.g. what is happening in the world outside). Clearly the content of the sessions also needs to be adapted to the functional levels of the group members.

In general, it is the effect of RO sessions rather than 24-hour RO that has been evaluated.[27] There is good support for the notion that certain aspects of cognitive functioning are enhanced by RO sessions, and especially performance on tests of orientation. It is less clear that any more generalised improvements in cognitive abilities of more general functioning occur without any special training in the aspect of behaviour of concern.[30] Another limitation is that any gains for RO disappear once the sessions are withdrawn.

Other special techniques are reminiscence therapy and validation therapy.[27,31] The former is based on the notion that older people tend to reminisce, and there is a rationale for the use of memories from the past in that people with dementia can recall things from the distant past whereas they may not be able to remember what happened yesterday. Talking about the past in a group setting can then be used as a bridge to discuss issues relating to the present.

Validation therapy grew out of the belief of an American social worker (Naomi Feil) that RO and similar methods were too confrontational and led to the person withdrawing and possibly becoming hostile. This could well be at least as much a criticism of the routine and unthinking way in which interventions like RO have been applied in some settings as being necessary aspects of the techniques themselves. Validation therapy stresses the validation of feelings in whatever time or place appears to be real to the individual, regardless of whether this corresponds to what staff members regard as the 'here and now'. The widow who talks as if her husband is still alive may be responded to not by denying this but, for example, by pointing out that the listener is aware that she was very fond of her husband.

In terms of evaluation, reminiscence therapy is less well explored than RO, but the evidence of any kind of potentially beneficial outcome is not great. There do appear to be changes within sessions,[27] but these have not been shown to be manifest outside the sessions. Validation therapy has yet to be properly evaluated. Possibly its greatest benefit is to remind staff that apparently disordered utterances need to be handled sensitively.*

This brief discussion does not exhaust the list of approaches that have been specially developed for use in dementia. Dementia care mapping[32] is one approach that has attracted much interest in the UK, although it so far has less to say as a specific approach to intervention as opposed to a way of assessment or evaluating quality of care. One key feature of all approaches mentioned in this section as well as some others which have not been mentioned is worthy of comment. Although they can be varied to suit the needs of individuals, they are all based, implicitly or explicitly, on a particular assumption about the nature of a key problem in dementia (e.g. loss of orientation in RO). A contrary point is that people with dementia do vary quite considerably and that what is the key problem (or set of problems) for one individual with dementia might not be the key problem(s) for another. In consequence, what are also required are methods of tackling problems relevant to individuals, and it is with such methods that the next section is concerned.

Interventions for individual problems

As already argued, people with dementia are different from one another and often have their own particular problems or difficulties, some of which may be amenable to psychological interventions. One class of such problems are those often referred to as 'challenging behaviour'.[33] Examples of challenging behaviour are aimless wandering, hoarding, refusing to bathe or wash, and so on.

Interventions to deal with such problems need to be specially designed on an individual basis in order to match the intervention to the nature of the problem, the characteristics of the individual concerned and the circumstances in which the problem arises. A wide range of potentially useful forms of intervention have been developed by clinical psychologists for use with other clinical groups, but which can be readily exploited and adapted to deal with the behavioural problems presented by those who suffer from dementia. These include such things as the behavioural and cognitive therapies.[25,34] However, these are best employed when the problem concerned has been subject to a careful functional analysis to determine the factors that enhance or reduce it.[35] Other means of ensuring that interventions match the needs of the individual

---

* Editors' note. The latest systematic review in the Cochrane Database finds insufficient evidence from randomised controlled trials to allow any conclusion about the efficacy of validation therapy for people with dementia or cognitive impairment.[37]

involved, such as analysing the problem graphically and evaluating the therapy process with the individual, have also been described.[36] There is evidence that such methods can be adapted successfully in work with those with dementia and that they can achieve at least some therapeutic goals.

General comment on interventions

The emphasis on developing psychological interventions for older people with dementia has been very much dominated by methods for use primarily in residential care settings, although there have been very occasional exceptions.[1] Given that a large proportion of those with dementia live in the community, often with some sort of support from relatives, more effort needs to be put into developing methods that can be used in the community. A useful model comes from the field of learning disability where a large literature has developed on ways of helping and training relatives (often parents) to develop simple strategies for themselves to deal with problems raised by severely learning-disabled family members.

CONCLUSIONS

This chapter has provided a brief outline of the contribution that psychological methods can make to the assessment and management of the person with dementia. Work in this area has become a rapidly expanding field. This chapter has set out to describe in outline some of the basic issues and space has precluded the detailed exploration of many aspects. This is especially so with regard to currently ongoing developments in the area of psychological interventions. The role of psychological assessment in dementia is much better established and this makes it easier to offer a reasonably definitive summary of this aspect.

Since dementia is biologically determined and progressive, it is clear that what can be achieved by psychological interventions alone is going to be limited. Nevertheless there is now good evidence that psychological or psychosocial interventions can at least help to maintain functioning and/or retard its decline. With recent and ongoing developments in the pharmacological treatment of dementia, the role of psychological interventions is likely to become enhanced. If pharmacological agents can slow down or even halt the underlying pathological process, this means that it is likely that those who suffer from dementia will tend to remain mildly impaired for much longer. Other forms of intervention, such as those of a psychological nature, that can help such people live as fully and independently as possible will then need to be used in tandem with pharmacological treatments if the overall quality of life of sufferers is to be maximised.

Key points

➤ Psychological assessment can make a useful contribution in the diagnosis of dementia, but like other methods for detecting dementia is not wholly accurate, and so evidence from psychological assessments needs to be considered in the context of other possible indicators.

➤ Within psychological forms of assessment, tests of memory offer the best single indicator of the presence of dementia.

➤ Psychological assessment is not very useful for discriminating between different forms of dementia.

➤ There is good evidence that even people with quite marked levels of dementia are sensitive to environmental influences. For example, even such simple things as the arrangement of furniture can have an effect on the amount of verbal interaction between residents in a residential unit.

➤ A number of specially designed forms of intervention for use with those suffering from dementia have been devised. The best known and best validated of these is reality orientation, but even here the gains are limited and short-lived after the programme has been discontinued.

➤ Special forms of intervention, such as reality orientation and reminiscence therapy, tend to assume that all those suffering from dementia share a single key disability or feature. This assumption may not be entirely true and the use of more specific forms of psychological intervention of the kinds used with other client groups should be considered in order to address the specific problems of individuals.

REFERENCES

1 Miller E, Morris R. *The Psychology of Dementia*. Chichester: John Wiley & Sons; 1993.

2 Miller E. The assessment of dementia. In: Morris RG (ed). *The Cognitive Neuropsychology of Alzheimer-type Dementia*. Oxford: Oxford University Press; 1996.

3 Hale WE, Stewart RE, Moore MT, *et al*. Electrocardiographic changes and cognitive impairment in the elderly. *Journal of Experimental and Clinical Gerontology*. 1992; **14**: 91–102.

4 Folstein MF, Folstein SE, McHugh PR. Mini-Mental State: a practical method for grading the cognitive state of the patient for the clinician. *Journal of Psychiatric Research*. 1975; **12**: 189–98.

5 Teng EL, Chui HC, Schneider LS, *et al*. Alzheimer's dementia: performance on the Mini-Mental State Examination. *Journal of Consulting and Clinical Psychology*. 1987; **55**: 96–100.

6   Wechsler D. *Wechsler Adult Intelligence Scale III*. San Antonio, TX: Psychological Corporation; 1997.

7   Nelson H, O'Connell A. Dementia: the estimation of premorbid intelligence using the new adult reading test. *Cortex*. 1978; **14**: 234–44.

8   Crawford JR. Current and premorbid intelligence measures in neuropsychological assessment. In: Crawford JR, Parker DM, McKinlay WW (eds). *A Handbook of Neuropsychological Assessment*. Hove: Lawrence Erlbaum; 1992.

9   Morris RG, Kopelman MD. The neuropsychological assessment of dementia. In: Crawford JR, Parker DM, McKinlay WW (eds). *A Handbook of Neuropsychological Assessment*. Hove: Lawrence Erlbaum; 1992.

10 Wechsler D. *Wechsler Adult Intelligence Scale III*. San Antonio, TX: Psychological Corporation; 1997.

11 Warrington EK. *Recognition Memory Test*. Windsor: NFER-Nelson; 1984.

12 Wilson B, Cockburn J, Baddeley AD. *The Rivermead Behavioural Memory Test*. Reading: Thames Valley Test Co.; 1985.

13 O'Brien JT, Beats B, Hill K, *et al*. Do subjective memory complaints precede dementia? A three-year follow-up of patients with 'benign senescent forgetfulness'. *International Journal of Geriatric Psychiatry*. 1992; **7**: 481–6.

14 Coslett HB, Saffran EM. Visuospatial functioning. In: Morris RG (ed). *The Cognitive Neuropsychology of Alzheimer-type Dementia*. Oxford: Oxford University Press; 1996.

15 Emery VOB. Language functioning. In: Morris RG (ed). *The Cognitive Neuropsychology of Alzheimer-type Dementia*. Oxford: Oxford University Press; 1996.

16 Miller E. Language impairment in Alzheimer-type dementia. *Clinical Psychology Review*. 1989; **9**: 181–95.

17 Warrington EK, McKenna P. *Graded Naming Test*. Windsor: NFER-Nelson; 1983.

18 Benton AL, Varney NR, Hamsher K. Visuospatial judgement: a clinical test. *Archives of Neurology*. 1978; **35**: 364–7.

19 Roth M, Tym E, Mountjoy CQ, *et al*. CAMDEX: a standardised instrument for the diagnosis of mental disorder in the elderly wit special reference to the early detection of dementia. *British Journal of Psychiatry*. 1986; **149**: 698–709.

20 Copeland JRM, Dewey ME, Griffith-Jones HM. A computerised diagnostic system and case nomenclature for elderly subjects: GMS and AGECAT. *Psychological Medicine*. 1986; **16**: 89–99.

21 Blacker D, Albert MS, Bassett SS, *et al*. Reliability and validity of NINCDS-ADRDA criteria for Alzheimer's disease. *Archives of Neurology*. 1994; **51**: 1198–204.

22 McKhann G, Drachman D, Folstein M, *et al*. Clinical diagnosis of Alzheimer's disease: report of the NINCDS-ADRDA Work Group under the auspices of the Department of Health and Human Services Task Force on Alzheimer's Disease. *Neurology*. 1984; **34**: 939–44.

23 Miller E. Some basic principles of neuropsychological assessment. In: Crawford JR, Parker DM, McKinlay WW (eds). *A Handbook of Neuropsychological Assessment*. Hove: Lawrence Erlbaum; 1992.

24 Kuriansky JB, Gurland BJ. The performance test of activities of daily living. *International Journal of Aging and Human Development*. 1976; **7**: 343–52.

25 Kazdin AE. *Behavior Modification in Applied Settings*. Homewood: The Dorsey Press; 1975.

26 Sommer R, Ross H. Social interaction on a geriatric ward. *International Journal of Social Psychiatry*. 1958; **4**: 128–33.

27 Woods RT. Psychological 'therapies' in dementia. In: Woods RT (ed). *Handbook of the Clinical Psychology of Ageing*. Chichester: John Wiley & Sons; 1996.

28 Lord TR, Garner JE. Effects of music on Alzheimer patients. *Perceptual and Motor Skills*. 1993; **76**: 451–5.

29 Cleary TA, Clamon C, Price M, *et al*. A reduced stimulation unit: effects on patients with Alzheimer's disease and related disorders. *Gerontologist*. 1988; **28**: 511–14.

30 Hanley IG, McGuire RJ, Boyd WD. Reality orientation and dementia: a controlled trial of two approaches. *British Journal of Psychiatry*. 1996; **138**: 10–14.

31 Woods RT. Cognitive approaches to the management of dementia. In: Morris RG (ed). *The Cognitive Neuropsychology of Alzheimer-type Dementia*. Oxford: Oxford University Press; 1996.

32 Kitwood T. Towards a theory of dementia care: the interpersonal process. *Ageing and Society*. 1993; **13**: 51–67.

33 Stokes G. Challenging behaviour in dementia: a psychological approach. In: Woods RT (ed). *Handbook of the Clinical Psychology of Ageing*. Chichester: John Wiley & Sons; 1996.

34 Woods RT. *Psychological Problems of Ageing: assessment, treatment and care*. Chichester: John Wiley & Sons; 2000.

35 Sturmey P. *Functional Analysis in Clinical Psychology*. Chichester: John Wiley & Sons; 1996.

36 Petermann F, Muller JM. *Clinical Psychology and Single-case Evidence: a practical approach to treatment planning and evaluation*. Chichester: John Wiley & Sons; 2001.

37 Neal M, Barton Wright P. Validation therapy for dementia. *Cochrane Database Syst Rev*. 2003; **3**: CD001394.

CHAPTER 6

The role of the physician for the elderly in the assessment, diagnosis and treatment of patients with dementia

Michael Carpenter and Abbie Flinders

INTRODUCTION

Dementia is a heterogeneous group of diseases that places a heavy burden on health and social services and especially informal carers. Patients with dementia have often been seen as a lost cause because of the incurable nature of the disease. However, incurable does not mean untreatable.

Treatment can ameliorate some of the symptoms for a proportion of sufferers, at least temporarily. There are secondary prevention strategies that may delay the progression of some of the underlying diseases. Patients with the so-called reversible dementias may potentially have their symptoms improved. Early diagnosis allows the timely input of advice and support, for sufferers and carers can often maintain the patient in their own environment.[1] All clinicians who manage patients with dementia should therefore recognise the importance of a formal diagnosis, a full management plan and attention to the small but significant factors that may improve the quality of life of the patient and their carers.

Patients with dementia usually present to the physician with previously unrecognised cognitive impairment in need of a diagnosis, or as a patient referred with another condition, the management of which may be affected by their dementia. Many patients present as an acute medical admission with a preliminary diagnosis of 'failure to cope', and are frequently mislabelled as social problems. There is an overlap because patients with dementia admitted to hospital may not have been diagnosed or fully assessed prior to admission.

A detailed discussion of the aetiology and diagnostic criteria for dementia is outside the scope of this chapter and has already been considered. However, one cannot discuss the management of these patients without reference to the diagnostic features of the different dementias.

REVERSIBLE DEMENTIA SYNDROMES

There are a number of illnesses that may be associated with a dementia-like picture. If the underlying condition is treatable, and treatment may produce an improvement in cognitive function, a missed diagnosis represents a lost opportunity to prevent dementia. This fear has led physicians to place an inordinate emphasis on diagnosing the reversible dementias.

In reality this group is very small and may have diminished further in recent years.[2] The cost-effectiveness of screening for the group is not clear.[2,3] An added complication is that many of the conditions are also accepted causes of acute confusional states. It is possible that any improvement in cognitive function of patients treated for reversible dementia may be due to the treatment of an acute confusional state superimposed on an underlying dementia. The most commonly involved diseases are listed in Box 6.1.

Box 6.1   Causes of reversible dementia

➤ Hypothyroidism
➤ Vitamin B$_{12}$ deficiency
➤ Folate deficiency
➤ Neurosyphilis
➤ Normal pressure hydrocephalus
➤ Frontal meningioma
➤ Hyperparathyroidism

Hypothyroidism

The diagnosis of myxoedema madness is old and predates any form of biochemical testing for hypothyroidism or curative therapeutic options. Several studies have shown improvements in cognitive functioning following treatment with L-thyroxine, but the degree of recovery is inconsistent and cure seems to be the exception rather than the rule.[4,5] Subclinical hypothyroidism detected on opportunistic testing may correlate with impaired cognition, with some studies showing that therapy leads to an improvement in cognitive function[4] with treatment. However, further randomised controlled trials with standardised measures of cognition and thyroid function are needed to clarify the matter.[6]

Older people are more prone to developing primary hypothyroidism[5] and signs and symptoms are often non-specific even in patients without cognitive impairment. Physicians should therefore routinely check thyroid function of elderly patients with an unexpected decline, physical or cognitive, particularly if it has not been checked in the last 12 months.

Vitamin B$_{12}$ deficiency

Vitamin B$_{12}$ deficiency is common in the elderly population with prevalence between 10% and 15% and males are more commonly affected than females.[7] The clinical signs – polyneuropathy and sub-acute combined degeneration of the spinal cord – are often not present in the elderly.[7] Haemopoietic effects also tend to be minimal with up to a third of patients showing no evidence of anaemia.[8,9]

Screening for B$_{12}$ deficiency is controversial as low levels do not necessarily reflect actual deficiency and normal levels may not exclude it.[7] Additionally, a significant proportion of patients with low B$_{12}$ will be missed if the mean corpuscular volume (MCV) alone is used to guide testing.[10] Serum homocysteine and methylmalonic acid levels have been suggested as additional measures but are not routinely used in clinical practice at this time.[7]

Epidemiological data exists to suggest a link between vitamin B$_{12}$ deficiency and cognitive impairment but a recent Cochrane Review surmised that studies have failed to show a significant improvement following treatment with cobalamin.[7] This may be a result of study design and it has been suggested that a time limit exists during which treatment could be beneficial.[11,12]

Folate deficiency

The association between folate deficiency and cognitive impairment is equally complicated. Weight loss and poor nutritional status commonly associated with dementia along with its complex interactions with homocysteine and vitamin B$_{12}$ make it difficult to study. However, a recent literature review suggests that low folate levels are consistently associated with poorer cognitive function on testing.[13] A subsequent study found that lower baseline folate levels were associated with a higher rate of incident dementia and new onset dementia was more common in those with a decline in folate levels over a 2.4-year time period.[14]

Syphilis

There is a significant debate about routine serological testing for syphilis for patients with cognitive impairment.[15–19] Less than 5% of elderly patients have positive serological tests on admission to hospital[15,20,21] and neurosyphilis as a cause of cognitive impairment is rare, tending to appear as isolated case reports.[17] Two large studies have found less than 1% of cases of potentially reversible dementia to be due to central nervous system syphilis.[2,16] In another large case series, almost all of the cognitive impairment was felt to be due to either Alzheimer's disease or cerebrovascular disease, with serological screening picking up coincident syphilis.[20]

Serological testing is complex due to the varying sensitivity of each test at different stages of the disease as well as false positive and negative results. Non-treponemal tests (e.g. venereal disease research laboratory, VRDL) alone are no longer recommended and either treponemal enzyme immunoassay or a combination of the two is now suggested.[22] For a diagnosis of active neurosyphilis, cerebrospinal evidence of syphilis is required.[23] This may be very difficult in frail patients, especially if they are likely to be restless during the procedure.

It is suggested that the test works better to 'rule in' rather that 'rule out' neurosyphilis[24] and that even with a positive result treatment may not be recommended.[15] Investigation for neurosyphilis should therefore only be carried out in those with clinical features to suggest the diagnosis.

Normal-pressure hydrocephalus

The classical presentation of normal-pressure hydrocephalus (NPH) is with a triad of gait apraxia, urinary incontinence and cognitive decline.[25] In practice, diagnosis is difficult. CT brain scan shows a dilated ventricular system with no effacement of the sulci. A similar pattern may be seen in small vessel disease, causing periventricular ischaemia with atrophy of the white matter resulting in expansion of the ventricles. Even though ischaemic changes are usually visible within the white matter in the latter, it can still be very difficult to distinguish the two.[26]

Following an evidence-based review, a group of neurosurgeons have proposed guidelines to assist in accurate diagnosis of NPH.[26] They suggest grouping patients into 'probable', 'possible' or 'unlikely NPH' categories based on history, specific clinical findings, brain imaging and CSF studies. The hope is to provide more consistency in diagnosis in future clinical trials.

The importance of accurate diagnosis is that treatment with ventricular shunt insertion carries a risk of significant morbidity (e.g. shunt infections, blockage), with up to 50% of patients requiring shunt revision at some stage.[27] Trials of shunt insertion show a wide range of results, in part due to the variations in outcome measures used and there are currently no randomised controlled trials comparing outcomes of shunt insertion versus no shunt.[28]

Selection of those patients who will benefit from the procedure has not produced clear guidance. Further investigations such as the lumbar tap test, prolonged external lumbar drainage and determination of the CSF outflow resistance via an infusion test can increase predictive accuracy.[29] Outcomes tend to be better in those with milder symptoms of a shorter duration.[30]

In summary, with no single diagnostic test and surgical intervention with uncertain outcomes, careful assessment is required before embarking on treatment.

Hypercalcaemia

Hypercalcaemia may be associated with a number of neuropsychological disturbances. Significant hypercalcaemia may result in a delirium responsive to lowering the serum calcium. The role of hyperparathyroidism in dementia has more recently been questioned. Some report dramatic improvements in cognition following parathyroidectomy despite serum calcium levels within normal limits.[31] However, a more extensive review of the literature found studies of cognition pre- and post-parathyroidectomy reported inconsistent findings.[32]

Summary

The diagnoses historically called reversible dementias are a small group of conditions, for which treatment can at best be expected to improve rather than cure cognitive impairment. Many of the investigations such as thyroid function, B vitamins and serum calcium are entirely reasonable to carry out in a frail elderly person presenting with new symptoms. However, other investigations should be directed by thorough history and clinical examination leading to a suspected diagnosis, rather than in routine screening. It is reasonable, therefore, to concentrate on better diagnosis and management of the common dementias, rather than diverting too much time and attention to the reversible forms.

ASSESSMENT AND DIAGNOSIS

The physician for the elderly has an important role in making the diagnosis of a dementia syndrome. Dementia care in the UK is most commonly managed by psychiatry-led memory services. However, dementia may be unrecognised at presentation or delirium considered, so patients may be first diagnosed by the physician.

It is not uncommon to find that dementia is the underlying diagnosis for patients referred because of falls, decreasing mobility, difficulty coping or even weight loss. It is therefore mandatory to carry out an assessment of cognitive function as part of any review of an older patient presenting with non-specific symptoms.[19] It is obviously important to consider other causes of these symptoms even when it is clear that the patient has a previously undiagnosed dementia.

The patient's perception of forgetfulness is not as reliable as the carer's perception, so corroborative evidence is vital.[33] Evidence of cognitive impairment does not in itself diagnose dementia. The history of onset, duration and progression of the forgetfulness, and any associated features, is needed. If the onset is acute, or the symptoms have been fluctuating, any history of changes in conscious level must be sought out. This is particularly important when patients are admitted acutely to hospital with confusion as there is often co-existent delirium and dementia.[34]

Other salient features in the history include the presence of symptoms such as speech difficulties, motor problems or dyspraxias. The presence of speech disorders, such as non-fluent dysphasia, dysarthria or echolalia, may suggest underlying cerebrovascular disease or a fronto-temporal dementia. The latter are more commonly associated with a younger onset.

A history of myoclonic jerks, cerebellar dysfunction and a rapid decline may suggest Creutzfeldt–Jakob disease (CJD). The sporadic variety is more common in older people and the BSE-related variant CJD is more common in younger people. The doctor should also ask about symptoms of thyroid disorders, though the classical symptoms are often absent in older people.

Examination of a patient with suspected dementia should be thorough. General examination should include looking for the peaches and cream complexion of the hypothyroid facies, along with bradycardia and slow relaxing reflexes. The physician should also look specifically for pyramidal signs to suggest anterior circulation stroke, or signs such as lead-pipe rigidity and postural instability that may indicate basal ganglia strokes.

Parkinson's disease (PD) should be considered if there is a pill-rolling tremor, cog-wheel rigidity, bradykinesia or other features such as micrographia. It is unusual for dementia to develop before the physical symptoms in PD.

Blood pressure measurement is required, especially if the patient's dementia turns out to have a vascular origin as hypertension should be one focus of secondary prevention.

A full medication review should take place, including over-the-counter products, with the aim of identifying and reducing the use of those that may adversely affect cognition.[35]

Investigations should include a search for common physical illnesses and include estimation of haemoglobin, urea and electrolytes, glucose, thyroid function, calcium, vitamin B_{12} and folate levels. If delirium is a possibility, a mid-stream urine sample should be taken and chest X-ray considered as clinically indicated. An ECG is useful as the presence of left ventricular hypertrophy indicates a higher risk of cerebrovascular disease.

Further investigation of the potentially reversible dementias should be considered as detailed previously.

All patients with suspected dementia should have brain imaging to aid diagnosis. Ideally this should be MRI but this will depend on local availability and CT scanning can also be used.[35] The presence of focal ischaemic changes will suggest a vascular basis for the disease, although co-existent Alzheimer's disease (AD) cannot be excluded. Excessive global cerebral atrophy is not diagnostic on a single scan but supports a diagnosis of AD in a patient with a consistent history. The presence of localised atrophy in the frontal and temporal lobes suggests a fronto-temporal dementia.

Where the primary diagnosis is unclear, referral to a neurologist for further assessment and investigation should be considered. A suspected diagnosis of CJD, for example, will require an EEG, MRI and lumbar puncture after discussion with the CJD surveillance centre in Edinburgh.

TREATMENT

The National Institute for Health and Clinical Excellence (NICE) recommends that acetylcholinesterase inhibitors are only started by specialists in the care of people with dementia, which includes elderly care physicians.[35] The effectiveness of treatment must be regularly reviewed using formal assessment methods.[35] Appropriate support for patients and family must be provided, either through community psychiatric nursing services or voluntary agencies such as the Alzheimer's Society. The complexities of management mean that an organised service is required and most physicians will therefore generally refer patients to a memory service for treatment.

If the diagnosis is vascular dementia the physician should consider secondary prevention strategies. There is currently no clear evidence that aspirin delays the progression of vascular dementia;[36] however, it is reasonable to extrapolate from the evidence for stroke disease. If the brain imaging shows evidence of cerebral infarction then clopidogrel 75 mg daily should be given, otherwise aspirin 75 mg daily would be a logical choice as many patients will have a history of ischaemic heart disease.

There is no clear evidence that treatment of hypertension prevents dementia in those without prior cerebrovascular disease.[38] The Hypertension in the Very Elderly Trial (HYVET), although finding no significant difference in the treatment groups alone, did find a borderline significant pooled ratio in favour of treatment when combined with other large studies.[39] Patients were not excluded from the HYVET if they had a history of previous cerebrovascular disease.

The PROGRESS collaborative group specifically selected patients who had had either a stroke or transient ischaemic attack (TIA) in the last five years. Treatment with perindopril with or without indapamide significantly reduced the risk of further stroke events.[40] The secondary end point of reduced risk of developing dementia only reached significance in patients who suffered a further vascular event while in the trial.[41] Further trials are needed for secondary prevention specifically in those with a diagnosis of vascular dementia. However, in view of the evidence in large vessel disease it would seem reasonable at this time to optimise blood pressure management in patients with vascular dementia.

Studies looking at the treatment of hypercholesterolaemia have generally focused on primary prevention of dementia. Statins in prevention of AD had initially looked promising. However, a recent Cochrane Review has concluded that statins given to individuals in later life at risk of vascular disease have no effect in preventing AD or other forms of dementia.[37]

Any co-existing medical conditions should be appropriately treated to reduce the disease burden.

Finally, but perhaps most importantly, the physician has a duty to discuss the diagnosis with the patient and their carers. At present only about one-third of patients with dementia are given a formal diagnosis during their illness.[1] In light of the different treatments and secondary prevention strategies available, giving patients the specific diagnosis is now a prerequisite of good care. Patients should be given appropriate verbal and written information on prognosis and treatment options. Time should be set aside for this and a suitable adult, usually the patient's next of kin or main carer, should be present.

Case Study 6.1

An 88-year-old woman was admitted from home after a fall. Examination revealed significant cognitive impairment, with an Abbreviated Mental Test score (AMTS) of 3/10, but was otherwise unremarkable. Routine investigations revealed marked hypothyroidism and she was commenced on replacement therapy immediately.

A history from her informal carer subsequently revealed increasing forgetfulness for many months, to the extent of leaving pans on the cooker to burn dry or lighting the gas cooker and hanging wet towels over it to dry.

Over the following six weeks her thyroid function returned to normal and her cognitive function improved. Her AMTS rose to 7/10, indicating persistent cognitive impairment. She remained incontinent of urine despite regular toileting and denied this was a problem. She was assessed at home but still lacked the ability to carry out simple domestic tasks, requiring frequent prompting, and was unaware of the risks she was taking.

Following a care planning meeting she was discharged to residential home and referred to the memory clinic for further assessment and follow-up.

DEMENTIA AND ACUTE ADMISSION TO A GENERAL HOSPITAL

Dementia is common amongst older patients admitted to hospital. Currently up to 70% of acute hospital beds are occupied by older people and it is thought that up to half may have either dementia or delirium.[1] It is not uncommon for the dementia to be undiagnosed[1] and therefore assessment of the mental state of all older people admitted to hospital is essential.

The most commonly used assessment tool validated in the hospital setting is the Hodkinson's Abbreviated Mental Test.[42] However, there may be inconsistencies in the questions asked between doctors using the tool.[43] A further problem with cognitive screening tools is the cultural unfairness of many of the tests.[44] Specific language versions of the AMTS and MMSE have been validated,[45,46] but increasingly there is a move toward culture-free tests.[44]

The 6CIT is one such test that is validated[47,48] and can be easily translated at the time of use. It is now being used increasingly in primary care settings and there will no doubt be a move toward this type of screening test in the hospital setting in the near future.

A collateral history is also an essential part of the acute assessment process. Very often a patient presents with an acute confusional state and only after careful discussions with family or carers does the history of increasing forgetfulness over many months become apparent. Personal experience suggests that relatives do not always equate confusion and forgetfulness and will deny any confusion but offer that the patient has been forgetful. They interpret confusion as an acute delirious reaction with disruptive behaviour.

It is important to recognise that many patients with dementia often exhibit a significant worsening of their cognitive function when acutely ill. The physician must make every effort to exclude an acute, treatable pathology. Dementia sufferers with an intercurrent illness often present with very vague symptoms and a trawl of the simple investigations such as a blood screen, urine culture, chest X-ray and ECG is required. A review of the medication is mandatory. All drugs likely to have a negative effect of cognitive function should be discontinued if safe to do so.

Many patients with dementia become acutely confused and disorientated after admission to hospital. They are five times more likely to develop delirium than patients without dementia.[49] The noisy environment, with constant changes of personnel and frequent ward moves, is probably the worst way to manage a confused patient. Patients should be managed wherever possible in a quiet area, with only familiar visitors in the early stages. There is evidence that using a multi-component approach to hospitalised elderly people may reduce the risk of delirium and shorten its course.[50]

The physician should resist the temptation to restrain or sedate patients and take a lead role in educating junior medical and nursing staff as to the reasons. The Royal College of Nursing offers specific guidance on restraint.[51] The Mental Capacity Act 2005 requires us to use the least possible restrictive method when treating or caring for a person who lacks capacity for that intervention.[52]

Over-sedation will render the patient unable to care for themselves. In hospital, these patients spend longer in bed and have longer lengths of stay. In a nursing home, they are more prone to infections and consume more resources from carers. Patients who exhibit signs of paranoia or extreme agitation may require sedation for short periods. Haloperidol or lorazepam should be used, offered orally first and given in the lowest effective dose.[35]

Attempting to restrain confused patients will often result in a breakdown in the patient–professional relationship, fostering paranoia and worsening disruptive behaviour. Cot-sides for beds will not prevent confused patients from wandering. Instead, they simply provide an extra means of accidental injury. Alarms for beds or seats may help ward staff to monitor the situation, but ideally patients should be allowed to roam in a safe environment. This is difficult in an acute hospital due to the number of critical areas the patient can invade, as illustrated by the Case Study 6.2.

Case Study 6.2

A 55-year-old woman with a diagnosis of Alzheimer's disease was admitted to a general ward after becoming unresponsive. She was mute with generalised increased tone, a temperature of 38°C and a mildly raised creatine kinase. She was taking haloperidol and the dose had recently been increased when she became disruptive whilst in respite care during a family holiday.

The haloperidol was stopped and her condition settled, with no cause for her pyrexia being found. A diagnosis of neuroleptic malignant syndrome was considered not proven, but the decision was made to avoid further exposure.

When she recovered she was very restless and would not sit in her chair. When left to wander she was at risk through inquisitive behaviour. She was constantly opening cupboards and interfering with equipment such as the cardiac defibrillator. She would frequently try to dance with frail patients, causing them to fall. Attempts to restrain her often produced a violent reaction.

An extra member of staff was assigned to walk with her and her behaviour became more manageable by diverting her attention away from critical situations without attempting to restrain her. The patient slept poorly, so the staff member was required 24 hours a day.

Patients with dementia provide a number of other challenges to hospital staff. The UK National Service Framework for Older People[53] requires that patients with mental health problems in acute general hospitals are cared for by staff with appropriate training. Patients with dementia have the right to be treated with the same respect as all other patients. Very often they may exhibit a stereotypical behavioural trait, such as echolalia or perseveration of speech. Healthcare workers should restrain the impulse to caricature such patients or encourage regressive behaviour.

Particular attention should be given to encouraging patients to eat and drink because malnutrition and dehydration have been highlighted as particular problems.[1] In the UK, training about this is ongoing through the Dignity in Care campaign.[54]

The physician may commonly find that a patient's cognitive function hinders their treatment due to lack of ability to consent or lack of compliance. All doctors should be able to assess capacity to consent, and this should be done on a decision-specific basis. The Mental Capacity Act 2005 is clear that we must not assume patients with dementia lack capacity.[52] If the patient is unable to consent the physician should look for alternative sources of consent. For instance, the patient may have an advanced directive for certain decisions and where this is legally recognised and valid it must be adhered to. Alternatively, the patient may have nominated another person using a lasting power of attorney for health and welfare decisions or there may be a court-appointed deputy. No one else can consent for a patient.

If there is no such person, the physician is able to treat in the patient's best interests. The physician should seek advice from relatives or close friends as to any previous wishes the patient has expressed. Most importantly, the physician must take into account the consequences of forcing the patient to have the treatment or test. For instance, sedation or even anaesthesia might be required to carry out a CT scan if the patient is unable to co-operate. This would add a significant risk of morbidity, and perhaps mortality, to the procedure and judgements about the risks and benefits of the test would clearly need to take that into account. For life-altering decisions a 'best interests' meeting should be convened to ensure that all aspects are properly considered.

At the extreme of refusal to consent, the patient may not take sufficient food and fluid to maintain their health. In such circumstances the physician should exclude physical reasons, such as oro-pharyngeal conditions, as well as considering co-existent depression or paranoia. Psychiatric advice may be needed. If no treatable cause is found, a detailed discussion with the family should be undertaken so that they understand the issues.

A more common problem in geriatric medicine is the patient with advanced dementia who develops neurologic dysphagia. This situation poses the difficult question of artificial feeding. Initially, attempts should be made to alter the consistency of food and supervise feeding. If this fails then the patient's individual circumstances should be carefully assessed by a multidisciplinary team, including discussions with the family about their views and whether the patient had previously expressed an opinion on this matter.

There is currently no evidence to suggest that enteral tube feeding is beneficial in patients with advanced dementia.[55] Nasogastric and percutaneous endo-scopic gastrostomy (PEG) feeding may be associated with a higher incidence of aspiration and shorter life expectancy.[56] The need for enteral feeding in itself may indicate a poor prognosis, with one UK study suggesting a 30-day mortality of 54%, rising to 78% at three months.[57] Offering appropriately thickened fluid and softened food in frequent, small amounts is associated with weight gain, and this may be the most appropriate course of action.

Finally, patients with dementia often cause difficulty when it comes to planning discharge. They require a more careful assessment because of the unreliability of self-reported abilities. Objective measures such as kitchen assessments and home visits by a occupational therapist can provide vital information regarding both patient safety and orientation within their usual environment. Compliance with medication is a common problem that may be addressed by the use of calendar packs and monitoring by carers. Drugs that have a narrow therapeutic index, such as warfarin, should be carefully considered to ensure the benefits outweigh the risks.

Even if assessments go well, carers and relatives may still have concerns regarding discharge. Planning at an early stage allows these concerns to be raised and provides an important opportunity to recognise carer strain, which could lead to elder abuse if not attended to. It has also been recognised that failure of communication between hospital teams and primary carers at the time of discharge leads to defective post-discharge management and potential readmission.[1] New roles such as discharge facilitators and mental health teams within the hospital should improve this over time.

Key points

➤ Older people presenting with a history of gradual physical decline should have their cognitive function assessed routinely.
➤ People with undiagnosed dementia often present to the physician with another unrelated condition.
➤ There is no evidence to support the cost-effectiveness of routine screening for the so-called reversible dementias in the absence of clinical indications.
➤ There are no controlled clinical trials to support treatment of an underlying cause of reversible dementias, but observational studies suggest improvement rather than cure.
➤ Patients with dementia in a general hospital often pose significant problems and are entitled to have access to appropriate expertise in their assessment and management.

> ➤ Capacity to consent should be considered at all times on a decision-specific basis without the assumption that it is lacking.
> ➤ Dysphagia in patients with dementia requires a full multidisciplinary assessment.
> ➤ Artificial feeding carries a high risk of morbidity and mortality in patients with dementia; regular feeding with small amounts of food and fluid of correct consistency may be a more appropriate management plan.
> ➤ Patients with dementia should have an objective assessment of their ability to manage at home prior to discharge from hospital.

REFERENCES

1 Department of Health. *Living Well with Dementia: A National Dementia Strategy.* London; 2009. Available at: www.dh.gov.uk/en/Publicationsandstatistics/Publications/PublicationsPolicyAndGuidance/DH_094058 (accessed May 2011).

2 Clarfield AM. The decreasing prevalence of reversible dementias. An updated meta-analysis. *Archives of Internal Medicine.* 2003; **163**: 2219–29.

3 Weytingh MD, Bossuyt PMM, Van Creval H. Reversible dementia. More than 10% or less than 1%. A quantitative review. *Journal of Neurology.* 1995; **242**: 466–71.

4 Bégin ME, Langlois MF, Lorrain D, *et al.* Thyroid function and cognition during aging. *Current Gerontology and Geriatrics Research.* 2008; Vol. 2008: Article ID 474868 doi:10.1155/2008/474868.

5 Dugbartey AT. Neurocognitive aspects of hypothyroidism. *Archives of Internal Medicine.* 1998; **158**: 1413–18.

6 Villar HCCE, Saconato H, Valente O, *et al.* Thyroid replacement for subclinical hypothyroidism. *Cochrane Database Syst Rev.* 2007; **3**: CD003419.

7 Malouf R, Sastre AA. Vitamin B_{12} for cognition. *Cochrane Database Syst Rev.* 2003; **3**: CD004394.

8 O'Broin SD, Kelleher BP, McCann SR, *et al.* The value of the erythrocyte indices as a screening procedure in predicting nutritional deficiencies. *Clinical and Laboratory Haematology.* 1990; **12**(3): 247–55.

9 Stott DJ, Langhorne P, Hendry A, *et al.* Prevention and haemopoietic effect of low serum vitamin B_{12} levels in geriatric medical patients. *The British Journal of Nutrition.* 1997; **78**(1):57–63.

10 Oosterhuis WP, Niessen RW, Bossiyt PM, *et al.* Diagnostic value of the mean corpuscular volume in the detection of vitamin B_{12} deficiency. *Scandinavian Journal of Clinical and Laboratory Investigation.* 2000; **60**(1): 9–18.

11 Abyad A. Prevalence of vitamin B_{12} deficiency among demented patients and cognitive recovery with cobalamin replacement. *The Journal of Nutrition, Health and Aging.* 2002; **6**(4): 254–60.

12 Martin DC, Francis J, Protech J, *et al.* Time dependency of cognitive recovery with cobalamin replacement: report of a pilot study. *Journal of the American Geriatrics Society.* 1992; **40**: 168–72.

13 Raman G, Tatsioni A, Chung M, *et al*. Hetergeneiry and lack of good quality studies limit association between folate, vitamins B-6 and B-12, and cognitive function. *The Journal of Nutrition*. 2007; **137**: 1789–94.

14 Kim JM, Steward R, Kim SW, *et al*. Changes in folate, vitamin B12 and homocysteine associated with incident dementia. *Journal of Neurology Neurosurgery and Psychiatry*. 2008; **29**: 864–8.

15 Boodhoo JA. Syphilis serology screening in a psychogeriatric population. Is the effort worthwhile? *British Journal of Psychiatry*. 1989; **155**: 259–62.

16 Rabins PV. Reversible dementia and the misdiagnosis of dementia: A review. *Hospital and Community Psychiatry*. 1983; **34**(9): 830–5.

17 Polsky I, Samuels S. Neurosyphilis: screening does sometimes reveal and infectious cause of dementia. *Geriatrics*. 2001; **58**(3): 61–2.

18 Kabasakalian A, Finney GR. Neurobiology of dementia chapter 15: Reversible dementia. *International Review of Neurobiology*. 2009; **84**: 283–302.

19 Siu AL. Screening for dementia and investigating its causes. *Annals of Internal Medicine*. 1991; **115**: 122–32.

20 Corrado OJ, Bowie PCW, Bagnall WE, *et al*. The prevalence of positive serological tests for syphilis among elderly hospital patients. *Age and Ageing*. 1989; **18**: 407–10.

21 Wooley PD, Anderson AJ. Prevalence of undiagnosed syphilis in the elderly. *Lancet*. 1986; **ii**: 1034.

22 Egglestone SI, Turner AJL. Serological diagnosis of syphilis. *Communicable Disease and Public Health*. 2000; **3**: 158–62.

23 Bowie PCW, Corrado OJ, Waugh MA. Screening for syphilis. *British Journal of Psychiatry*. 1990; **156**: 283–4.

24 Dans PE, Cafferty L, Otter SE, *et al*. Inappropriate use of the cerebrospinal fluid venereal disease research laboratory (VRDL) test to exclude neurosyphilis. *Annals of Internal Medicine*. 1986; **104**: 86–9.

25 Warrell D, Cox T, Firth J, *et al*. *Oxford Textbook of Medicine*. Oxford: Oxford University Press; 2004.

26 Relkin N, Marmarou A, Klinge P, *et al*. Diagnosing idiopathic normal-pressure hydrocephalus. *Neurosurgery*. 2005; **57**(3 Suppl.): S2–16.

27 Pujari S, Kharkar S, Metellus P, *et al*. Normal-pressure hydrocephalus: long-term outcome after shunt surgery. *Journal of Neurology Neurosurgery and Psychiatry*. 2008; **79**: 1282–6.

28 Esmonde T, Cook S. Shunting for normal pressure hydrocephalus. *Cochrane Database Syst Rev*. 2002; **3**: CD003157.

29 Marmarou A, Bersgsnieder M, Klinge P, *et al*. The value of supplemental prognostic tests for the preoperative assessment of idiopathic normal-pressure hydrocephalus. *Neurosurgery*. 2005; **57**(Suppl. 2): S17–28.

30 Peterson RC, Mokri B, Laws ER, Jr. Surgical treatment of idiopathic hydrocephalus in elderly patients. *Neurology*. 1985; **35**: 307–11.

31 Papageorgiou SG, Christou Y, Kontaxis T, *et al*. Dementia as a presenting symptom of primary hyperparathyroidism: Favourable outcome after surgery. *Clinical Neurology and Neurosurgery*. 2008; **110**: 1038–40.

32 Coker LH, Kashemi R, Cantley L, *et al*. Primary hyperparathyroidism, cognition and health-related quality of life. *Annals of Surgery*. 2005; **242**(5): 642–50.

33 McGlone J, Gupta S, Humphrey D, *et al*. Screening for early dementia using memory

complaints from patients and relatives. *Archives of Neurology.* 1990; **47**: 1189–93.

34 Kolbeinsson H, Jónsson Å. Delirium and dementia in acute medical admissions of elderly patients in Iceland. *Acta Psychiatr Scand.* 1993; **87**: 123–7.

35 National Institute for Health and Clinical Excellence. *Dementia. The NICE-SCIE guidance on supporting people with dementia and their carers in health and social care. NICE guideline 42.* London: NICE. www.nice.org.uk/guidance/GC042

36 Rands G, Orrell M, Spector AE. Aspirin for vascular dementia. *Cochrane Database Syst Rev.* 2000, 4: CD001296.

37 McGuinness B, Craig D, Bullock R, *et al.* Statins for the prevention of dementia. *Cochrane Database Syst Rev.* 2009; **2**: CD003160.

38 McGuinness B, Passmore T, Bullock R. Blood pressure lowering in patients without prior cerebrovascular disease for prevention of cognitive impairment and dementia. *Cochrane Database Syst Rev.* 2006; **2**: CD004034.

39 Peters R, Beckett N, Forette F, *et al.*, for the HYVET investigators. Incident dementia and blood pressure lowering in the Hypertension in the Very Elderly Trial cognitive function assessment (HYVET-COG): a double-blind, placebo controlled trial. *Lancet Neurology.* 2008; **7**(8): 683–9.

40 PROGRESS collaborative group. Randomised trial of a peridopril-based blood-pressure-lowering regimen among 6105 individuals with previous stroke or transient ischaemic attack. *Lancet.* 2001; **358**(9287): 1033–41.

41 PROGRESS collaborative group. Effects of blood pressure lowering with peridopril and indapamide therapy on dementia and cognitive decline in patients with cerebrovascular disease. *Archives of Internal Medicine.* 2003; **163**: 1069–75.

42 Qureshi KN, Hodkinson HM. Evaluation of a ten-question mental test in the institutionalized elderly. *Age and Ageing.* 1974; **3**: 152–7.

43 Holmes J, Gilbody S. Differences in use of abbreviated mental test score by geriatricians and psychiatrists. *British Medical Journal.* 1996; **313**: 465.

44 Parker C, Philp I. Screening for cognitive impairment among older people in black and minority ethnic groups. *Age and Ageing.* 2004; **33**: 447–52.

45 Rait G, Burns A, Baldwin R, *et al.* Validating screening instruments for cognitive impairment in older South Asians in the United Kingdom. *International Journal of Geriatric Psychiatry.* 2000; **15**(1): 54–62.

46 Rait G, Morley M, Burns A, *et al.* Screening for cognitive impairment in older African-Caribbeans. *Psychological Medicine.* 2000; **30**(4): 957–63.

47 Brooke P, Bullock R. Validation of the 6 item cognitive impairment test. *International Journal of Geriatric Psychiatry.* 1998; **14**: 936–40.

48 Davis PB, Morris JC, Grant E. Brief screening tests versus clinical staging in senile dementia of the Alzheimer's type. *Journal of the American Geriatric Society.* 1990; **38**: 129–35.

49 Royal College of Physicians. *The Prevention, Diagnosis and Management of Delirium in Older People.* Concise guidance to good practice no 6. London: RCP; 2006.

50 Inouye SK, Bogardus ST, Jr, Charpentier PA, *et al.* A multicomponent intervention to prevent delirium in hospitalized older patients. *New England Journal of Medicine.* 1999; **340**(9): 669–76.

51 Royal College of Nursing. *Let's Talk About Restraint.* London: RCN; 2008.

52 Mental Capacity Act 2005. Available at: www.legislation.gov.uk/ukpga/2005/9/contents (accessed May 2011).

53 Department of Health. *National Services Framework for Older People.* London: DoH; 2001. Available at: www.dh.gov.uk/en/publicationsandstatistics/publications/ publicationspolicyandguidance/DH_4003066 (accessed May 2011).

54 Social Care Institute for Excellence. *Dignity in Care.* Adults' services guide 15. London: SCIE; 2009.

55 Sampson EL, Candy B, Jones L. Enteral tube feeding for older people with advanced dementia. *Cochrane Database Syst Rev.* 2009; **2**: CD007209.

56 Finucane TE, Christmas C, Travis K. Tube feeding in patients with advanced dementia. *Journal of the American Medical Association.* 1999; **282**: 1365–70.

57 Sanders DS, Carter MJ, D'Silva J, *et al.* Survival analysis in percutaneous endoscopic gastrostomy feeding: a worse outcome in patients with dementia. *American Journal of Gastroenterology.* 2000; **95**: 1492–5.

CHAPTER 7

The general practitioner's perspective

Linda Harris (revised for this edition by John Wattis)

INTRODUCTION

The National Service Framework (NSF) for Older People[1] was published in 2001 and followed in 2009 by a National Dementia Strategy for England[2] and corresponding strategies or plans for Wales, Scotland and Northern Ireland. The NSF was a big step forward in attaching government priority to the health-care of older people. It was based around standards and charged local health and social care organisations with putting in place a systematic and sustainable programme by which the standards would be implemented for all old people, whether at home, in a residential setting or in hospital. There were four themes in the NSF:

➤ rooting out age discrimination
➤ providing person-centred care
➤ promoting older people's health and independence
➤ fitting services around people's needs.

The NSF specifically addressed those conditions which are particularly significant for older people, such as stroke, falls and mental health problems associated with old age (with a focus on depression and dementia). Of course, these conditions are not exclusively problems of old age and so the principles applied to all age groups. The National Dementia Strategy, published in 2009 after wide consultation, stated its purpose was to:

- Provide a strategic quality framework within which local service can deliver quality improvements to dementia services and address health inequalities relating to dementia

- Provide advice, guidance and support for health and social care commissioners ... [and providers] in the planning, development and monitoring of services and

- Provide a guide to the content of high-quality health and social care services for dementia to inform the expectations of those affected by dementia and their families.

It has three broad themes: raising awareness and understanding, early diagnosis and support and living well with dementia. There are also 17 detailed objectives (*see* Box 7.1), most of which have direct implications for GPs and others in primary care. Following the publication of the White Paper, *Equality and Excellence: liberating the NHS*,[3] with its radical restructuring of the commissioning and provision of healthcare, it is uncertain how far the strategy will be carried through. However, the basic principles of the National Institute for Health and Clinical Excellence (NICE) setting standards and the Care Quality Commission inspecting quality will remain. At present there are estimated to be around 700 000 people in the UK with dementia.[2] The rise in the numbers of elderly people, especially the 'very old', means that GPs are finding themselves managing an increasing number of people with dementia. In Europe, dementia is more common than stroke in terms of both incidence and prevalence; but mental illness, especially dementia and depression, goes unrecognised in primary care.[4]

Box 7.1 The objectives of the National Dementia Strategy for England

1 Improving public and professional awareness and understanding of dementia.
2 Good quality early diagnosis and intervention for all.
3 Good quality information for those with diagnosed dementia and their carers.
4 Enabling easy access to care, support and advice following diagnosis.
5 Development of structured peer support and learning networks.
6 Improved community personal support services.
7 Implementing the carers' strategy.
8 Improved quality of care for people with dementia in general hospitals.
9 Improved intermediate care for people with dementia.

10 Considering the potential for housing support, housing-related services and telecare to support people with dementia and their carers.
11 Living well with dementia in care homes.
12 Improved end-of-life care for people with dementia.
13 An informed and effective workforce for people with dementia.
14 A joint commissioning strategy for dementia.
15 Improved assessment and regulation of health and care services and of how systems are working for people with dementia and their carers.
16 A clear picture of research evidence and needs.
17 Effective national and regional support for the strategy.

Nearly 20 years ago, the journal *Geriatric Medicine* surveyed 500 GPs from a random sample of 1500 readers and found that six out of ten GPs found Alzheimer's disease very difficult to manage and eight out of ten felt there were insufficient resources locally to help them deal effectively with this group of patients.[5] Just over 10 years ago, the Audit Commission produced its *Forget Me Not* report into mental health services for older people.[6] This was followed by the NSF[1] and the National Dementia Strategy,[2] already mentioned. It is still unclear how far these worthy documents have positively influenced developments.

The age-related prevalence of dementia, coupled with the increasing numbers of elderly people raises difficult questions about causes and treatment. However, in responding to the management of the problem , health and social commentators advocate an holistic approach that will help both sufferers and their carers to bear the *burden* of dementia.

Not surprisingly, it is the strengths of general practice as the patient's advocate and the gateway to services that is so central to the care of this group of patients.

THE ROLE OF THE GP IN THE EARLY STAGES OF THE DISEASE

> Only 31% of GPs believe they have received sufficient basic and post-qualification training to diagnose and manage dementia, a decrease since the same question was asked in the Forget Me Not report eight years ago.
>
> (National Dementia Strategy,[2] p. 26)

People with dementia and those caring for them often first seek help from their GP. It is clear that the GP and the primary healthcare team (PHCT) have a key role in the early stages of the disease, providing information, support and competent advice. The Dementia Strategy[2] says that early diagnosis not just of dementia but of the *subtype* of dementia should be made by a specialist as part of a specially commissioned service (p. 37).

With the availability of effective treatments for dementia, it is crucial that an early diagnosis is made so that anti-dementia drugs are made available (alongside other early interventions) for those people who meet the criteria published by NICE. Despite this, only about a third of people with dementia receive a formal diagnosis at any time in their illness and a number of secondary healthcare and social services staff have expressed concerns over the delay in some GPs identifying mental health problems, with situations often reaching a crisis point before specialist mental health services are alerted.

GETTING GPS INVOLVED IN TREATING THE PHYSICAL AS WELL AS THE MENTAL HEALTH NEEDS OF PATIENTS EXHIBITING EARLY SIGNS OF DEMENTIA

> When dementia is suspected and once acute confusional states and other conditions requiring urgent action have been excluded, the patient should be referred to a specialist service for early diagnosis (National Dementia Strategy.[2] p. 35).

One of the challenges of working with older people is the frequency with which diseases present in a non-specific way. This is particularly the case in people with dementia. The only safe rule in practice is always to suspect underlying physical illness in old people presenting with increased confusion (or other psychiatric syndromes). History remains undeniably the most important way of gleaning information from the patient; but for completeness and in the case of an acute or chronic confusional state an increasing number of key people need to be consulted, such as relatives, the warden, the home help, neighbours and district nurses (within the reasonable bounds of confidentiality).[7]

The causes of acute, subacute and chronic disease states are dealt with elsewhere in this book and there are a large number of physical conditions that produce at least some of the clinical features of dementia, such as restlessness, impaired concentration, emotional lability and behavioural deterioration. It is important that GPs conduct a careful assessment and medical examination and give such patients the benefit of the doubt as well as their knowledge, avoiding the all too common conclusion that dementia or 'senility' is entirely to blame.

When a physical diagnosis is made, the primary aim is to ensure that any physical illness is treated as quickly and effectively as possible, that efforts are made to ease pain and discomfort and that an early review of medication is made. Patients with confusional states related to physical problems often require help from specialists in both the medicine and psychiatry of old age; and throughout the process information, advice and counselling for relatives will need to be provided by the GP.

The good GP will also be aware that carers for people with dementia themselves often suffer physical and mental distress and illness. The carer may neglect their own physical health needs because of the pressure of caring and for fear of what will happen to their loved one if they need hospital treatment for themselves. Carers also become depressed more often than those not carrying the burden of caring.

WHERE DEMENTIA AND DEPRESSION CO-EXIST

The prevalence of depression in patients with dementia is around 20% and, in some settings, up to 10% of patients initially thought to have organic dementia are later diagnosed as having depression or depressive pseudodementia.[8]

For busy GPs, distinguishing between depression and dementia can be difficult. However, with careful assessment it is usually possible. Interestingly, the skills involved in unravelling this diagnostic conundrum illustrate the close relationship between depression and cognitive impairment and ensure that both of these conditions are considered carefully in terms of the most appropriate assessment and management plan to be applied by the GP and PHCT. Box 7.2 lists some of the points to consider when managing patients with depression.

Box 7.2   Depression and dementia[8]

➤ Most patients with dementia are not depressed
➤ Most patients with depression are not demented
➤ Even when the two are found together, one usually predominates
➤ Remember to assess both memory and mood in elderly patients
➤ Depression often responds to antidepressants, even in dementia

---

Cognitive impairment secondary to depression

Those elderly patients whose depressive illness is associated with profound psychomotor retardation, apathy, loss of motivation and slowed thought processes may perform poorly on bedside tests, wrongly suggesting a diagnosis of dementia. Many depressed old people fail to keep up with basic self-care and lose weight, such that a dementia may be strongly suspected and a depressive illness may be overlooked.

Depression secondary to cognitive impairment

Depression in patients with dementia may have a psychological or organic cause. In early dementia, sufferers may retain sufficient insight to be distressingly aware of the loss of their valued intellectual abilities. Even more devastating will be the effects of their knowledge and understanding of the progressive nature of the disease, which is associated with increased suicide risk.

As dementia progresses, a patient's insight becomes impaired, leading to increased disappointment, sadness and frustration at their failures at everyday tasks and loss of independence. In addition, organic brain disease may lead directly to low mood by affecting neuro-endocrine regulation or to an apathetic state that mimics true depression.

Factors leading to both depression and dementia

Various drugs and illnesses can cause both depression and cognitive impairment. One of the most important is alcohol. Whilst alcohol abuse is less prevalent in advanced old age, it can cause both depression and memory problems, with the potential to cause permanent memory dysfunction and dementia.[9] It is important, therefore, to consider alcohol abuse in the elderly and a simple questionnaire such as CAGE or the AUDIT questionnaire should facilitate further discussion in the consultation.[10] Drugs such as L-dopa, indomethacin, furosemide, steroids and many others may cause depression or delirium, especially in those with pre-existing organic brain disease.

Some diseases can precipitate either depressive or cognitive symptoms or both; these include Parkinson's disease, hypothyroidism and strokes. There are, of course, cases of coincidental co-morbidity where the two disorders occur together by chance and the longitudinal relationship evolves such that the earliest symptom of depression is cognitive impairment (or vice versa).

TIPS ON RECOGNITION AND MANAGEMENT OF PATIENTS IN PRIMARY CARE WHERE THE DIAGNOSIS BETWEEN DEMENTIA AND DEPRESSION IS UNCLEAR OR WHERE THERE IS A COMBINATION OF DEPRESSION AND COGNITIVE IMPAIRMENT

The most important diagnostic aid is the history from both patient and, where possible, a reliable informant. Enquire about the onset and duration of symptoms and about other illnesses, drugs taken and alcohol. Certain features are linked more with depression or pseudo-dementia. These include:

➤ relatively short duration between onset and consultation
➤ previous psychiatric history
➤ a more precise date of onset of symptoms
➤ they are more likely to complain of poor memory and to be self-critical

➤ they are more likely to answer 'I don't know'
➤ recent and remote memories appear equally impaired.

Good management is reliant upon the GP or PCHT member using a standard assessment tool such as the Abbreviated Mental Test (AMT) Score,[11] which is good at detecting significant cognitive impairment (*see* Box 7.3). Depression, on the other hand, is more easily overlooked, though a simple enquiry into the patient's mood, perhaps coupled with a standard mood questionnaire such as the Geriatric Depression Scale,[12] is extremely useful in determining the true underlying cause and thereafter the most appropriate care plan. Again, if dementia is suspected, the patient should be referred to a specialist service for (early) diagnosis and management.

It is important to consider mood, even in someone with established dementia, as depressive symptoms will often respond to antidepressants. It is important also to remember that even modest improvements in symptoms can make large differences to carers.

Box 7.3   Abbreviated Mental Test[11]

Each question scores one mark. No half marks. A score of 6 or less suggests dementia (or another cause of cognitive impairment).

1 Age
2 Time (to nearest hour)
3 An address (e.g. 42 West Street, to be repeated by the patient and recalled at the end of the test)
4 Year
5 Name of hospital, residential institution or home address of present location
6 Recognition of two people (e.g. doctor, nurse, relative, home help, etc.)
7 Date of birth
8 Year First World War started
9 Name of present monarch
10 Count backwards from 20 to 1

SHARING THE DIAGNOSIS WITH PATIENT AND CARER

… new, specialist services need to be commissioned to deliver good quality early diagnosis and intervention…They would provide an inclusive service, working for people of all ages and from all ethnic backgrounds. Their sole focus would be on early diagnosis and intervention for people with dementia. This would include:

- Making the diagnosis well:
- Breaking the diagnosis well to the person with dementia and their family: and
- Providing directly appropriate treatment, information, care and support after diagnosis.

(National Dementia Strategy,[2] pp. 36–7)

If the strategy is implemented, these specialist services will have the role of sharing diagnosis with the patient in the first instance. Memory clinics and memory services already perform this function for those referred to them. Whoever breaks the news, it is important that the GP and the PHCT are aware of what has been said and to whom. It is also important that there is locally shared information about prognosis, treatment and general support and how to access it so that all health and social care workers present accurate information to patients and carers.

THE CHALLENGES POSED BY ATTEMPTS TO MAINTAIN CONFIDENTIALITY AND AUTONOMY OF THE PATIENT

In the early stages, many patients resist proposed interventions and changes in their routines and there are clear obligations for the GP and the PHCT around patient confidentiality. Clearly, autonomy is to be encouraged, bearing in mind the limits of patients' abilities. Driving is one of the relatively few areas where it is appropriate for an official body to impose its judgement on both carer and patient.[13] In general, most decisions about management are best made by those most closely involved with the day-to-day life of the patient rather than by a committee of the courts. A balance must be struck between paternalistic care and naïve attachment to the patient's 'overriding right' to self determination. When dealing with the sensitive area of fitness to drive GPs will often refer to the regularly updated information published by the Driver and Vehicle Licensing Authority (DVLA) which contains helpful information and guidance.[14]

For many relatives this will be their first experience of the illogicality and inconsistency of dementia. Whilst the professional will know that pre-emptive action before a crisis occurs will usually result in a better outcome and improved quality of life, all too often there is difficulty in accepting the diagnosis, sometimes exacerbated by collusion (or conflict) between patient and partner. Ultimately, it is through open discussion of problems and possible solutions that optimum care can be achieved. Major management decisions can then be made collectively, by members of the PHCT and the family in consultation, as much as possible, with the patient. Occasionally, a consensus is difficult to achieve. The GP is then ideally placed to act as a moderator, balancing the background knowledge of patient and family with his or her own experience and expertise.[15]

MANAGING THE PATIENT WITH A DIAGNOSIS OF DEMENTIA WHEN SPECIALIST SERVICES HAVE TO BECOME INVOLVED

At present only a minority of patients with dementia are seen by specialist services, though coverage is improving. If the National Dementia Strategy is implemented nationally, then, ideally, all patients with suspected dementia will be referred for specialist diagnosis and early intervention. For the present this is not generally the case. At present the GP will make a judgement about when to call in specialist assessment, usually from a specialist memory service or perhaps from the community mental health team for the elderly. By this time the GP will have generally performed his or her own mental health assessment and will have looked carefully for any underlying physical illness, ordering simple 'baseline' investigations.

For patients to derive maximum benefit and for carers to be in a position to understand and offer support, then all the involved professionals need to exchange information and share decision making. The actual members of the PHCT involved and their core disciplines are less important than the systems they have set up to communicate between themselves and with other relevant groups, such as the memory service, the community mental health team and the local social services department.

The 2001 NSF demanded that a single assessment process be introduced for the health and social care of old people. The fact that the 2010 White Paper is still emphasising the need for close co-operation between health and social services suggests that the single assessment process has not been very successful.

The balance of provision of care for people with dementia is for home-based services, so the GP must remain in close contact with the family, the memory service, the community mental health team and any others involved. The PHCT can keep track of services that are put in place and ensure that the patient and carer are receiving services and support appropriate to their needs. Primary care practitioners realise just how much the burden of care falls on the relatives (and other 'informal' carers). Carers put up with many problems with good grace and are worn down by others (*see* Box 7.4).[16] They are central to the success of community care, but the personal costs to them are great and it is imperative that we support them.[17]

GPs have the key role of orchestrating the provision of diagnostic services, community support and institutional care of the highest standard. They feel confident in community services when they are provided sensitively and flexibly.

Box 7.4   Problems associated with caring for older people with significant mental morbidity[16]

Carers' problems – well tolerated
➤ Reduced social life
➤ Embarrassment
➤ Anxiety and depression
➤ Dressing
➤ Washing
➤ Urinary incontinence

Carers' problems – poorly tolerated
➤ Aggression
➤ Verbal abuse
➤ Wandering
➤ Faecal smearing
➤ Inappropriate urination
➤ Sleep disturbance
➤ Restless by day

Frustrations are experienced where there is limited access to memory services or multidisciplinary community mental health teams for the elderly. The core members of a specialist mental health service should include a consultant psychiatrist specialising in mental health problems in old age, community mental health nurses, clinical psychologists, occupational therapists and social workers. Home care workers should be trained in the provision of services to those with mental health problems. An agreed written care plan that is regularly reviewed and updated is essential to shared understanding between professionals, patients and carers.

GPs need to know that all of the above is in place and that in addition they can also access day-care places and respite care providing a range of stimulating and appropriate group and one-to-one activities to preserve the abilities of patients (so far as possible) and provide relief to carers. With these in place, GPs can more confidently support and encourage carers to continue caring and co-operating with home-based models of treatment.

MANAGING THE PATIENT WITH DEMENTIA WHO LIVES ALONE

Fortunately, the majority of Alzheimer's disease patients live with carers or have the benefit of carers' regular input. However, a small but significant minority live alone with little family support. This results in a potential for delayed diagnosis and failure to track deterioration in cognitive and physical function. The Alzheimer's Society, the World Health Organization and old age specialists have tried to encourage primary care-led 'over 75 health checks' to identify people with potential dementia who have nobody else to report their lapses of memory and difficulties with self-care.[18] This means going to the homes of those who have not attended the surgery recently and including in the examination some form of cognitive screening such as the AMT.[11]

Sadly, despite the drive to engage more GPs and their PHCTs in the early detection and monitoring of patients who have dementia and live alone, evidence suggests that GPs, overburdened with the responsibilities of meeting the growing needs of all their patients, will make no more house calls than absolutely necessary and rarely perform a cognitive test. It seems that they are sceptical of the benefits of early detection and fear the demands on their time. The whole system must acknowledge this and seek to engage PHCTs in this task so that they remain the focal point for care co-ordination.

THE GP AND THE PATIENT WHOSE CLINICAL CONDITION IS DETERIORATING

Finally, as the disease progresses, patients may no longer be in a position to cope at home and once again the GP may become involved in organising admission to hospital or a residential or nursing home. GPs can and should advocate for maintaining as many people as possible in their own homes in the community, provided any problems can be managed by community services without throwing an unacceptable strain on family carers.

Hospital admission should be avoided whenever possible. In an emergency, an inpatient psychogeriatric or geriatric admission, depending on the balance of behavioural and physical problems, may be necessary and should be the opportunity for a thorough and comprehensive review of care needs and how they can be met. On discharge the GP is often faced with a revised community care plan and changes to the patient's medications. The post-discharge visit is therefore vital to update the GP records and ensure that the GP and PHCT continuity of care is maintained. Sometimes a radical revision of the care plan may result in discharge to a residential or nursing care facility. There may often be a change of GP at this point for geographical reasons.

Out-of-hours services are becoming increasingly sophisticated with respect to the care of people with dementia. This is largely due to the development of care pathways supported by district nursing services and rapid response teams. Single assessment systems mean that increasingly a GP contacted out of hours can access a practitioner from rapid response who will arrange for the patient to be supported either in their own home with additional help or admitted to a short-term care facility. The GP will usually need to assess the patient first, to ensure any medical problems are identified and appropriately managed, then a contribution can be made to the overall assessment (including the assessment of risk) and a treatment plan can be developed. The increased emphasis on intermediate care services for people with dementia in the National Dementia Strategy[2] means that increasingly GPs will be able to use these for short-term care or to facilitate longer-term care in residential or nursing homes. Psychiatric services for old people have always had a strong community component and that is likely to need to develop further as the shift away from inpatient NHS care continues.

EDUCATION AND TRAINING FOR GPS AND PHCTS

This is in line with the first objective of the National Dementia Strategy (*see* Box 8.1). Surveys reported earlier in the Audit Commission's *Forget Me Not* report[6] showed that over 50% of GPs reported feeling insufficiently trained in the recognition and management of dementia. This had increased to nearly 70% by the time of the National Dementia Strategy[2] (p. 26). In contrast nearly two-thirds of GPs felt adequately trained in the diagnosis and management of depression. Training and support from local specialist mental health teams for the elderly, memory services and the proposed diagnostic and early intervention specialist teams seems to be the best way not only of increasing GP and PHCT education in this area but also of building bridges between the different components of the services.

Assessment scales like the AMT mentioned earlier help to ensure that cognitive impairment is not missed and that the diagnosis of dementia is considered. Despite this, the Audit Commission's surveys[6] showed that fewer than half of GPs were using specific screening tools or protocols to help diagnose depression or dementia.

The proposed GP commissioning consortia that will take on the commissioning role of existing primary care trusts (PCTs) will need to consider how and where to commission education for their own PHCTs to improve the quality of primary care for people with dementia (and other mental health problems in old age).

Under the regime of PCTs, protected learning time sessions have been developed, facilitated and funded through the PCT, which allow GP surgeries to close for one half day per month for training purposes. Education in dementia diagnosis and management is an obvious priority for such sessions and can be developed with the aid of local specialist teams. Indeed, there is a case for specialist teams being proactive in identifying practices with low referral rates and 'selling' appropriate training to them. All practice staff who engage clinically with older people should at least receive training in the recognition of dementia, delirium and depression and in the use of simple assessment scales for depression and cognitive impairment.

The use of scales such as the AMT or the longer Mini Mental State Examination for cognitive impairment and the GDS for depression can become part of standard care pathways for older people with mental health problems agreed between primary and secondary care services. Training is known to reap rewards and there is strong evidence linking the provision of training and the value placed by GPs on early detection.[19]

THE GP AND INFORMATION QUALITY AND CLINICAL AUDIT

Information to empower patients is one of the key planks of the White Paper, *Equality and Excellence*.[3] In the case of people with dementia, who may not be able directly to access and use the information for themselves, empowering family and other informal carers is equally important. 'Over-75 health checks' can be standardised and recorded electronically. Patients and carers can then (at least in theory) find out how well any GP practice performs in this task of monitoring the over-75 population. Referral rates to specialist memory services can also be monitored. Public health physicians can also in theory use this data to plot health needs and trends.

THE GP AND MEDICINES MANAGEMENT

For some time now GPs have been expected to review the medications for the over-75s on their lists at least every year. This is facilitated by computerised prescribing systems and often reviews are conducted every three or six months. Community pharmacists have an increasing role in helping older people to use their medications appropriately.

The gains for older people with mental health problems through medication review are many. They are the group most likely to be using four or more medications and most likely to need prescribing advice and support. Regular review by the GP improves the quality and cost-effectiveness of prescribing and helps avoid waste. Good practice in this area reduces adverse events, side effects and unwanted interactions, as well as reducing the risks of suicide in the depressed patient or accidental self-poisoning in patients with dementia. Particularly relevant for patients with dementia is the opportunity to eliminate inappropriate prescription of antipsychotics and long-term (ab)use of other sedatives for behaviour problems.

PREVENTION AND PROMOTING THE HEALTH OF THE PATIENT WITH DEMENTIA

Good medicines management is one very important way that a patient's health can be promoted. However, all older patients, regardless of cognitive function, have the right to the benefit of good advice and support in reducing risks to their physical and mental health. As the National Dementia Strategy[2] puts it succinctly, 'What is good for the heart is good for the head' (p. 27). Up to 50% of dementias have a vascular component and even 'pure' Alzheimer's disease may share some risk factors with vascular disease. Thus, measures to decrease the risk of cardiovascular disease and stroke are also relevant in dementia. On a much smaller but probably increasing scale, the avoidance of excessive alcohol consumption is also important. Good management of hypertension, the avoidance of obesity and adequate exercise also have a role to play, as do social interventions and other actions to alleviate the stress of carers.

Primary care is an important route of access to mainstream health promotion and disease prevention programmes. The PHCT, in particular the practice nurses, can advise patients and carers on the most appropriate actions around primary and secondary prevention or, more positively, around promoting optimal health. As well as cardiovascular health, dietary advice, attention to the prevention and management of osteoporosis, access to annual flu vaccination programmes and the prompt detection and management of chest and urinary infections all help promote better health for people with dementia and their carers.

CONCLUSIONS

We hope we have demonstrated how the GP and PHCT can become useful companions to people with dementia and their families on their journey of care. By walking the clinical path *with* the patient, the GP will remain in the best position to support the complex needs of both patients and their families.

Such complexity needs to be managed by co-ordination of health and social care through teams that provide an integrated service to the patient. Efforts to ensure effective information sharing, working alongside patients and a willingness to consult and/or visit them regularly means that the GP will continue to be central to the care planning of people with dementia.

With the ever-increasing pressure on primary care to improve standards, and now to take a more active role in commissioning services, a strong personal commitment is required of GPs and their teams to ensure that the needs of older people with dementia are not neglected.

Education and training from local memory services, services for early diagnosis and intervention in dementia and community mental health teams for older people will help to build bridges and equip PHCT members with the knowledge and skills to help them undertake their most important roles of early detection and monitoring.

By becoming involved proactively in the multidisciplinary management of dementia, the GP and practice team will be rewarded. Potential benefits include being able to deal competently with the increasing needs of patients in a timely, evidence-based manner, with the added bonus of seeing the carers (so often also our patients) gain the tangible benefits of integration into mainstream primary care services.

Carers need to be empowered to cope and patients need to know that their GP practice will support and facilitate their right to early assessment and equal access to the full range of physical and mental health services they deserve.

Clinical commissioning groups and health and well-being boards have a responsibility to bring together the necessary commissioning of health and social care in order to meet the holistic healthcare needs of patients and carers.

On 16 June 2011, The Royal College of General Practitioners launched a new educational programme, developed in partnership with the Department of Health, The Princess Royal Trust for Carers and with support from The Children's Society, to help GPs and primary care teams better support the growing number of people who care for others. The e-learning sessions include information about the valuable part that carers play in supporting some of the most vulnerable people in society, and the ways in which GPs and their teams can organise their practices and work with carers to achieve this. The sessions also incorporate information about carers' own health and information needs, the difficulties that they face in addressing these and possible ways in which the primary care team might help.

Key points

➤ GPs and nurses in the primary care team are recognised as having a crucial role in early detection of dementia and its successful management.

➤ Training for GPs and PHCT members in dementia management is vital to change attitudes and improve the early detection and co-ordinated management of dementia. This should concentrate on professional role, use of cognitive assessment tools and other strategies for early detection, good practice strategies, referral for early and accurate diagnosis, how to cope with difficult behaviour and how to access specialist support services.

➤ Many resources are required in dementia care, including clinical expertise from the doctor and an up-to-date, wide-ranging knowledge of local and regional resources (including the help available nationally and in many areas locally through the Alzheimer's Society). Any shortfalls in resource awareness will disadvantage patients and their families. In the case of dementia, the caring, interested GP is often best placed to oversee care and identify and plug any gaps or faults in the provision of care.

> ➤ NICE guidelines highlight the role of cholinesterase inhibitors in the treatment of patients with Alzheimer's disease of moderate severity. GPs need to be aware of care pathways that enable access to specialist memory services, and the referral should not be delayed till the dementia is obvious, since early detection has many benefits, aside from the relatively small benefit from the current generation of cholinesterase inhibitors.

REFERENCES

1 Department of Health. *National Service Framework for Older People*. London: DoH; 2001.

2 Department of Health. *Living Well with Dementia: a national dementia strategy*. London: DoH; 2009.

3 Department of Health. *Equality and Excellence: liberating the NHS*. London: DoH; 2010.

4 Jorm AF, Jolley D. The incidence of dementia: a meta-analysis. *Neurology*. 1998; **51**: 728–33.

5 Grace J. Alzheimer's disease: your views. *Geriatric Medicine*. 1993; **23**(1): 39–41.

6 Audit Commission. *Forget Me Not: mental health services for older people*. London: Audit Commission; 2000.

7 Eccles J, Wattis J. Underlying physical causes of confusion in the elderly. *Geriatric Medicine*. 1988; **18**(4): 55–63.

8 Rao R, Dening TR, Brayne C, *et al.* Suicidal thinking in community residents over eighty. *International Journal of Geriatric Psychiatry*. 1997; **12**: 337–43.

9 Black DA. Changing patterns and consequences of alcohol abuse in old age. *Geriatric Medicine*. 1990; **20**(1): 19–20.

10 DTB. Managing the heavy drinker in primary care. *Drugs and Therapeutics Bulletin*. 2000; **38**(8): 60–4.

11 Qureshi K, Hodkinson M. Evaluation of a 10-question mental test of the institutionalised elderly. *Age and Ageing*. 1974; **3**: 152–7.

12 Yesavage J. Geriatric Depression Scale (GDS): recent evidence and development of a shorter version. *Clinical Gerontology*. 1986; **9**: 165–73.

13 Oppenheimer C. Dementia and driving. In: Oppenheimer C, Jacoby R (eds). *Psychiatry in the Elderly*. Oxford: Oxford University Press; 1991.

14 Driver and Vehicle Licensing Authority. *At a glance guide to the current medical standards of fitness to drive*. Swnasea: DVLA: 2010 [cited 25 August 2010]. Available at: www.dft.gov.uk/dvla/medical/ataglance.aspx (accessed May 2011).

15 Jones RG. Ethical and legal issues in the care of demented people. *Reviews in Clinical Gerontology*. 1993; **3**: 55–68.

16 Argyle N, Jestice S, Brook CPB. Psychogeriatric patients: their supporters problems. *Age and Ageing*. 1985; **14**: 355–60.

17 Levin E, Sinclair I, Gorbach P. *Families, Services and Confusion in Old Age*. Aldershot: Avebury; 1989.

18 World Health Organization. Diagnosis and management of dementia in primary care. *Guidelines: Summary of Clinical Guidelines for Primary Care*. 2002; **16**(2): 164–6.

19 Renshaw J, Scurfield P, Cloke L, *et al.* General practitioners' views on the early diagnosis of dementia. *British Journal of General Practice*. 2001; **51**: 37–8.

CHAPTER 8

The role of the nurse in the assessment, diagnosis and management of patients with dementia

Richard Clibbens

INTRODUCTION

Nurses are in a powerful position to influence the care of people with dementia for good or ill. In primary care, hospital care, the care home sector and many other environments, nurses are at the heart of care and treatment for people with dementia. The richness of the nursing contribution to care can be compromised by a lack of insight, knowledge and communication skills, but awareness of the needs of people with dementia and confidence in providing high-quality nursing interventions can make a huge positive difference to the lives of people with dementia and their carers at all stages and in all environments. At any one time the majority of people with dementia are living at home, where their care is often led or delivered by families, neighbours, friends and unqualified care workers. Interventions by professionals must acknowledge this and do nothing to imperil or destroy existing, often complex, networks of support. Nurses have a vital role in supporting people with suspected dementia to access proper assessment and diagnosis. Early diagnosis and intervention can greatly assist in enabling the person with dementia and their family to plan for the future, make advanced decisions and cope more effectively with cognitive deterioration, through accessing appropriate timely information and support.

ASSESSMENT

Nurses have a vital and often central role in the assessment of people with dementia. The range of settings and opportunities for nurses to positively engage in these processes of assessment is diverse, ranging from general health screening with older people in primary care, through to specialist memory assessment clinics and myriad other clinical and care situations. Nurses working in general hospital settings and residential or nursing homes, for example, may be the key professional or named nurse co-ordinating the care of older people, in settings which are recognised to include a high prevalence of dementia: up to 70% of acute hospital beds are occupied by older people and up to half of these people may have cognitive impairment including those with dementia and delirium.[1] Poor care can lead to malnutrition and dehydration for people with dementia, in turn impacting on cognition, recovery and discharge.

The nursing role in assessment and diagnosis may be in providing a unique nursing perspective or in co-ordinating multidisciplinary assessment in addition to completing the core elements of a comprehensive person-centred assessment.

NICE (2006) has identified that a diagnosis of dementia should only be made after a comprehensive assessment, including a review of medication to identify and minimise the use of drugs that may affect cognitive function.[2] People should be asked if they wish to know the diagnosis and with whom this should be shared. Formal cognitive testing should be undertaken using standardised instruments such as the Mini Mental State Examination (MMSE) or 6 Item Cognitive Impairment Test (6-CIT).[2] While assessment scales can form a useful component of assessment, such as of baseline cognitive function, they are still only a part of the whole picture of that person's experiences and are not usually diagnostic in their own right.[3]

The potential roles and influence of nursing in the assessment of people experiencing dementia have been identified to include:

➤ being the 'main support' person
➤ independently assessing the person at home, in clinic or hospital
➤ history taking from the person and family
➤ administering psychological tests
➤ carrying out joint assessments with colleagues.[4]

People who are or may be experiencing dementia clearly require a full nursing assessment, in addition to a specific focus on their unique experience of dementia.

The 'Six Senses' framework (*see* Box 8.1) provides a model that describes the elements needed where care is provided for people with dementia and that sustains effective relationships between all involved.[5] In assessment, account

Box 8.1   The Six Senses

1   A sense of security

For older people: Attention to essential physiological and psychological needs to feel safe and free from threat, harm, pain and discomfort.

For staff: To feel free from physical threat, rebuke or censure. To have secure conditions of employment. To have the emotional demands of work recognised and to work within a supportive culture.

2   A sense of continuity

For older people: Recognition and value of personal biography. Skilful use of knowledge of the past to help contextualise present and future.

For staff: Positive experience of work with older people from an early stage of career, exposure to role models and good environments of care.

3   A sense of belonging

For older people: Opportunities to form meaningful relationships, to feel part of a community or group as desired.

For staff: To feel part of a team, with a recognised contribution, to belong to a peer group, a community of gerontological practitioners.

4   A sense of purpose

For older people: Opportunities to engage in purposeful activity, the constructive passage of time, to be able to achieve goals and challenging pursuits.

For staff: To have a sense of therapeutic direction, a clear set of goals to aspire to.

5   A sense of fulfilment

For older people: Opportunities to meet meaningful and valued goals, to feel satisfied with one's efforts.

For staff: To be able to provide good care, to feel satisfied with one's efforts.

6   A sense of significance

For older people: To feel recognised and valued as a person of worth, that one's actions and existence are of importance, that you 'matter'.

For staff: To feel that gerontological practice is valued and important, that your work and efforts 'matter'.

must be taken of the relationships and family dynamics, as carers may resist interventions which are interpreted as threatening to their 'normalisation'.

> ... a systematic approach to assessment is required in which strengths and positive factors are identified as well as hazards which pre-dispose people to risks in certain circumstances

> (Parsons,[6] p. 134)

Physical screening

Whether at the level of health screening in primary care, during hospital admission or in residential care settings, nurses, in collaboration with medical colleagues, must ensure that an appropriate initial physical assessment is carried out for people who may be experiencing dementia (*see* Box 8.2). This must include screening to exclude underlying physical illness or delirium. NICE guidance[7] on the diagnosis, prevention and management of delirium (2010) provides a useful 'decision tree' to be utilised when a person aged 65 or older presents to hospital or long-term care. Agreed local protocols for cognitive screening and initial assessment can assist in appropriate screening for and detection of dementia in primary care. This will usually include referral to local memory assessment services where dementia is suspected.

Box 8.2   Baseline investigations for dementia[2] (adapted)

➤ Routine haematology
➤ Biochemistry tests (including electrolytes, calcium, glucose, renal and liver function)
➤ Erythrocyte sedimentation rate or C reactive protein test.
➤ Vitamin B_{12} and folate
➤ Thyroid function tests
➤ Midstream urine test (if delirium suspected)
➤ ECG/chest X-ray if indicated by clinical presentation
➤ Structural imaging (MRI or CT)

SHARING THE DIAGNOSIS

Alzheimer's Disease International[8] has described the shock of a dementia diagnosis, emphasising the value of good, accurate information in assisting to resolve some of the anxiety at this time for the person and their family. Nurses can utilise their roles in a range of health settings to provide support, education and information at such critical times as these in the journey of dementia, for both the person and their family.

The nursing contribution to diagnosis sharing in dementia is often of vital importance.[4] Nurses are often well placed to have identified the person's wishes with regard to diagnosis disclosure over a period of time. This may include the identification of any conflict of interests in diagnosis sharing with the person's family. For example, a person experiencing memory impairment may fear being assessed as unfit to hold a driving licence following receipt of a dementia diagnosis, while their family may have concerns for their driving safety and view a diagnosis as enabling this situation to be managed.

The National Dementia Strategy[1] has identified that all people with dementia should have access to a pathway of care that delivers an accurate, sensitively delivered diagnosis. Treatment, care and support should be provided as needed after diagnosis. The NICE Dementia Quality Standards (2010)[9] identify that people with dementia should receive care from people appropriately trained in dementia care and identify the importance of ensuring that people with dementia and their carers access information about their condition and local support services. Following a diagnosis of dementia it is vital that people have time and support to consider:

➤ advance statements (which allow people to state what is to be done if they subsequently lose capacity)
➤ advance decisions to refuse treatment
➤ lasting power of attorney (a legal document allowing people to state in writing who they want to make certain decisions for them if they cannot make them for themselves, including about personal health and welfare)
➤ preferred priorities of care (decisions about future care choices and where the person would like to die).

It is important that people are not overloaded with information at the time of diagnosis, but equally that they have the opportunity to plan for the future while they retain the capacity to do so. Nurses must be familiar with the principles of the Mental Capacity Act 2005 to ensure that all decisions made on behalf of someone with dementia, where they lack capacity, are in their best interests and take their wishes and desires into account.[1]

Alzheimer's Disease International[8] has identified that listening to the person's 'story' of the development of dementia is the most important element of diagnosis. Nurses are often the members of the multidisciplinary team best placed to elicit and record the person's story, fulfilling a key role in accurate assessment and diagnosis. Nurses can combine this key role with a unique individual representation of that person and their personal history, translating the assessment process into a vehicle for recognition of the individual and validation of their personal and unique identity in the presence of dementia. At a time of potential great stress and anxiety, the nurse may be able to recognise the potential strategies and reactions of the person with dementia, who may appear resistive to the process of diagnosis and assessment.[10] Moniz-Cook[11] has described the use of individualised programmes for people in the earlier stages of dementia, which incorporate counselling for losses, reinforcement of coping strategies, crises prevention advice and memory management programmes, tailored to the specific needs of the individual. Many areas now provide group interventions for people with dementia post diagnosis and their carers to promote effective coping and future planning in the presence of dementia.

Information provision following diagnosis is crucial[2] and referral to organisations and services providing post-diagnostic support is a vital component of effective intervention. Increasingly 'memory cafes' and other recreational and support groups, with activities such as 'singing for the brain', art workshops or dance and movement workshops, offer a mixture of cognitive stimulation, physical activity and social stimulation that can all contribute greatly to the well-being of people with dementia. In many areas, local branches of the Alzheimer's Society and other carers' organisations host a range of support networks and groups for people with dementia and/or their partners so they can access information and peer support, sharing and learning from each other's experiences and supporting each other through the challenges that lie ahead.

INTERVENTIONS

Assessment is often the first of many interventions. Whether engaged in assessment and care planning in the earlier stages, or further through the person's individual journey of dementia, the nurse can have a key influence on how this is experienced by the person and their family;

> The key principles which emerge are concerned with ensuring that practice is undertaken within a person-centred, values based approach which sustains a focus on positive action and which actively works to ensure that dependency and negativity is always minimised. These principles are equally applicable across all stages in the process, across all professions and across service settings.
>
> (Stanley and Cantley,[12] p. 122)

Significant differences may exist between professional notions of assessment and diagnosis and that of the person with dementia and their family.[13] In recent years a number of studies have begun to explore the experience of dementia from the perspective of the person, and now people with dementia themselves are describing their experience of dementia in research studies exploring diagnosis disclosure.[14]

There are potential conflicts of interest in responding to the expressed views and wishes of the person with dementia and that of their carers or family. Identified differences of opinion must be objectively recorded within the assessment process, clearly identifying who has expressed them.

Cognitive stimulation

Cognitive stimulation has been identified as an intervention that can be tailored to someone with dementia's level of cognitive functioning and provided on an individual basis or in a group session to assist in stimulating and maintaining cognitive functioning.

An example of cognitive stimulation in practice[15]

In a group situation there is a game called 'famous faces' which aims to improve cognitive problem solving and communication. One person is not shown the famous name or picture but has to ask questions of the group such as 'alive or dead', 'man or woman' until eventually guessing the right one.

Life story work

Life story work is the collection of memories based on information about a person's life. It can enable individuals to relive events that are significant or important and enable the expression of preferences, familiar routines and choice. This can help support well-being and personhood for people with dementia and be a therapeutic process in itself.

Life story work can help shape a positive future, through using the past and present to develop and continue a person's life story. Understanding a person's history can help to make sense of the present and is of real value, however it is important to be mindful that it is a story and the story doesn't end with the 'here and now'. A person's life story should contain their wishes and aspirations for the future and it should grow, be ongoing and added to as required.[16]

Assessment of behaviour

The potential difficulties experienced by a person with dementia in social settings, such as a hospital ward or residential home, can lead to behaviour that may be described as 'challenging' or 'disturbed'. This may be related to a whole range of factors related to how that individual relates to people, their physical environment and also their internal perception and understanding of what they are experiencing. The potential loss of normal social inhibitions, problems in recognising people and their roles or difficulty understanding what is expected from them are some potential challenges for the person with dementia in relating to those around them. Behavioural changes and disturbance experienced by the person with dementia may have significant impact on carers and be a key element in placement decisions and planning the provision of care.[17]

The many potential losses experienced by a person with dementia entering a formal care setting, such as familiarity, independence, security, companionship or orientation, can potentially be profoundly distressing and associated with behaviour labelled as disturbed, especially in the presence of any impaired communication abilities. It may be difficult for the person with dementia to retain a sense of their unique identity in the presence of potential loss of skills and social roles, combined with anxiety or fear for their future.[18]

In assessing the behaviour of people experiencing cognitive impairment, the nurse will need to obtain an objective assessment of exactly what is occurring. This can be achieved by observing and accurately recording the following elements of what is often described as 'disturbed behaviour'.

➤ What were the Antecedents (what was happening immediately before the behaviour occurred)?

➤ What was the Behaviour (objective description of what the actual behaviour was, not interpretations of what the behaviour may mean)?

➤ What were the Consequences of the behaviour (what were the outcomes for the person and others)?

This information can be collected over time across the 24-hour care period and evaluated in the context of that person's unique identity and life history. It may be useful to consider a range of questions.

➤ Does the behaviour represent the psychological, physical or emotional expression of pain or distress?

➤ Is the person's previous ability to communicate verbally altered in the presence of dysphasia?

➤ Is the person experiencing sensory deficits?

➤ Does the behaviour occur at a particular time?

➤ Is it in response to a particular situation or person?

➤ Is it related to communication between the person and others?

➤ Is it related to care-giving interventions?

➤ Is it related to external stimuli in the environment?

➤ Is the person fulfilling a psychological/emotional/physical need by this behaviour?

It may often be possible to identify periods of time where a person needs more support. If, for example, a person with dementia in a medical ward becomes distressed each time their visitors leave, can their sense of possible isolation, loss or abandonment be made more bearable through engaging in a social intervention with nursing staff on the ward at the point at which their family depart?

With their detailed and often intimate care contact with people with dementia in formal care settings, nurses can utilise their knowledge of the person to plan individualised care and interventions to minimise many potential causes of reported behavioural disturbance.

Nurses have a vital role in ensuring that people with dementia are not inappropriately prescribed medicines such as benzodiazepines or antipsychotics as a first response to behaviour that is identified as problematic. The NICE dementia guideline (2006)[2] sets out clear guidance to be followed when prescribing these treatments for people with dementia, including identification of and quantification of the target symptoms to be treated and the requirement for these medicines to be regularly reviewed to identify whether they are well tolerated and providing continued benefit. The NICE guideline identifies that alternatives to the prescription of these treatments should be considered first to alleviate distress or reduce risk for people with dementia who are experiencing psychological or behavioural symptoms. Professor Banerjee's report *Time for Action* (2009)[19] has indicated that antipsychotic prescribing could potentially be inappropriate for one in three people with dementia currently prescribed this medication, particularly highlighting the need for care home staff to be trained and equipped with alternative approaches in the management of psychological or behavioural symptoms of dementia.[2,19]

Design

The design of care environments has a significant impact on the well-being and independence of people with dementia. The Scottish Intercollegiate Guidelines have identified measures that should be considered when planning an environment for people with dementia, including:

➤ incorporating small-size units
➤ separating non-cognitively impaired residents from people with dementia
➤ offering respite care as a complement to home care
➤ relocating residents, when necessary, in intact units rather than individually
➤ incorporating non-institutional design throughout the facility and in dining rooms in particular
➤ moderating levels of stimulation
➤ incorporating higher light levels
➤ using covers over fire exit bars and door knobs to reduce unwanted exiting
➤ incorporating outdoor areas with therapeutic design features
➤ making toilets more visible and easier to access.[20]

In relation to risk management with people with dementia, careful assessment and observation is essential.[21] The person's true ability to function in their own environment must be assessed and not their ability to function in the potentially disorientating environment of a hospital ward. This is essential when planning for discharge and the provision of care packages. Nurses acting as key workers for people with dementia have a vital role to ensure that effective multidisciplinary assessment has taken place at the right time, in the right environment to facilitate maintaining the person's optimum functioning.

CAPACITY

The word 'dementia' may instil a fear into the person to whom it is applied, that they are somehow necessarily less capable. Nurses have a vital role in ensuring that the person with dementia's right to consent to care and treatment is maintained. Where a person may lack capacity with regard to any element of independent decision making in relation to their health and social care, this must be formally assessed and comply with the requirements of the Mental Capacity Act 2005.[22] Clearly, each individual will experience dementia differently, with differing rates of progress of the condition and differing retained strengths and experienced losses. Too often the term dementia can still be interpreted to suggest some form of automatic loss of capacity. As nurses we must question 'who' is deciding 'what' is in the person's best interests, and on what basis. Nurses should inform people with dementia and their carers about advocacy and voluntary services and encourage their use.[2]

PERSON-CENTRED CARE

The extensive work related to personhood and dementia by authors such as Kitwood has, according to Adams,[23] done much to set dementia and its care within a moral framework which attributes value to people with dementia.

A nursing focus of care must be 'to assist sufferers and relatives to find meaning within the illness experience and to assist them to preserve, even during the final deterioration of the patient, a notion of personhood' (Box 8.3).[24]

Box 8.3   Six criteria for personhood[25]

1   Consciousness (particularly the capacity to feel pain)
2   Reasoning
3   Self-motivating activity (i.e. renewable behaviour driven from within)
4   The capacity to communicate
5   The presence of self-concept
6   Self-awareness

Nurses have a unique opportunity and responsibility to lead and influence the formal and informal care team in the establishment of person-centred care (Box 8.4). Regardless of the arena, diagnosis must build upon a skilled, informed and sensitive interpretation of assessment. This, in conjunction with a clinical diagnosis, must generate clear and specific statements that identify the person's and their families' actual and potential needs and retained strengths and abilities.

HOSPITAL ADMISSION

In 2009 the Alzheimer's Society report *Counting the Cost*[26] identified that hospitals were failing to provide acceptable standards of care for people with dementia. In 2010 the NHS Confederation report *Acute Awareness*[27] identified how hospital admission can lead to confusion and sometimes agitation for people with dementia, impacting on their physical and psychological health and leading to longer hospital stays. Improvements in hospital environments, dementia training for staff and clear dementia care pathways have been identified as key elements in improving the care of people with dementia in hospital and in supporting effective discharge planning that can prevent unnecessary readmission.

Box 8.4   Person centred care[28]

➤ Respect for personhood
➤ Valuing interdependence
➤ Investing in care giving as a choice

For many people with dementia admission to an acute general hospital is the event which exposes their experienced cognitive changes and it is essential that their independence is promoted and skills maintained to maximise opportunities for them to return home on discharge.[29] The following aspects of care are essential.

➤ Ensure people are supported to eat and drink if required. Do not assume the person understands what is expected of them when meals and drinks are provided.
➤ Prevent and pay attention to constipation.
➤ Assist and encourage the person to use the toilet. Some people may not recognise toilet signs or be able to recognise and verbalise their needs.
➤ Assist and encourage with personal hygiene and care.
➤ You may need to use different approaches. Seek advice from family or friends on the best approaches to use.
➤ Provide positive encouragement.

➤ Do not automatically correct people where this causes distress.
➤ Encourage achievable tasks to maintain skills and independence.
➤ Provide stimulation and interaction appropriate to the individual.
➤ People with dementia can become more disorientated at night. Ask about night-time routines and habits at home that may help them settle in the hospital.[29]

Diagnostic and therapeutic interventions in accident and emergency departments may stimulate behaviours in the patient which have been previously unseen or concealed by relatives. The ensuing concern and distress must be recognised and managed. Transfer to a ward area, therefore, may deliver a patient and family at their most vulnerable into an already busy clinical area. Interactions at this time may set inappropriate benchmarks upon which future actions and relationships are built. Tolson *et al.*[30] have described the potentially threatening nature of an acute ward environment and the feeling of worthlessness generated in both patients and visitors.

Tolson *et al.*[30] identify that acute nursing care is at its best when delivered in tandem with recognition of the special needs of the person with dementia. The recognition and planning of care for a person with dementia must be clearly translated into effective and consistent care delivery. Tolson has previously identified the historical lack of recognition of, or recording of assessments relating to, cognitive impairment in documentation within acute hospital settings.

Case Study 8.1   Mrs S

Mrs S has an established diagnosis of dementia, and has been supported in her own home by a complex network of lay and professional carers. The daughter of Mrs S leads family input. There have been growing concerns about the safety of Mrs S as she is becoming increasingly frail and she is discovered on the lounge floor at 8 a.m. by her daughter on her 'routine call' to give mum her breakfast prior to commencing work. Mrs S is cold, shocked and has obvious pain in her leg/hip, and an ambulance is called. Mrs S has fractured her femur and is 'fast tracked' on arrival at the hospital using an integrated care pathway designed to meet the immediate needs of a person suffering from a fractured neck of femur. Post operatively, Mrs S is withdrawn, drowsy and reluctant to take fluid or food. The briefest details were recorded prior to surgery, and the nurse who is leading the care of Mrs S now begins to establish 'who is this person', recording information from Mrs S where possible and from her daughter. The nutritional assistant has asked about her favourite food and drinks.

Her daughter states: 'They reminded me about her glasses, I had forgotten in the rush. They explained about the anaesthetic, pain tablets, change of environment and trauma before and after admission and how they may have effected Mum. This made me feel better. I thought I had "lost my Mum". The care plan was there for Mum and I to see, and the physiotherapist was so patient and knew Mum soon forgot her advice and gently reminded her. They asked us to bring family photographs for Mum's locker and I wrote down what time I would visit where she could see it. Mum had always been a very quiet person and since her illness was unlikely to instigate a conversation, but even on this busy ward I felt they cared about her and valued her enough to find out about her and I never felt she was "abandoned in the corner".'

Assessment of Mrs S's post-operative condition acknowledged that she may not demonstrate discomfort, pain, thirst, hunger, bladder or bowel problems in 'normal' ways, and skilled interventions ensured that these were identified and managed. Rehabilitation processes acknowledged her short-term memory loss, and skilled discharge planning built upon retained strengths and well-established support networks and ensured discharge was timely and well supported.

CARE HOMES

Up to 75% of residents in non-specialist care homes for older people have dementia, and the prevalence rises to between 90% and 100% in homes with specialist dementia registration.[19] There are care homes that provide excellent care for people with dementia and the characteristics of such homes have been described:

> They generally pay close attention to leadership and staff management, staff training and development, and person-centred care planning. They also provide a physical environment that enables people with dementia to move around the home freely but safely. They provide purposeful activities that relate to individual preferences as well as general entertainment, and actively involve relatives and friends in the care of residents. They include a therapeutic approach in their nursing model and promote social interaction with staff at times other than when personal care is being delivered. They develop strong links with, and involvement in, their local communities and effective links with local healthcare services, including with specialist old age psychiatric services. They have a strong view of the resident as an individual with a set of past experiences which can form

the basis for communication and the development of relationships. Equally, such homes seek out and enable the provision, within the home, of therapeutic activities such as art therapy, music therapy or dramatherapy, which may enhance the social environment and the possibility for self-expression.[19]

The Alzheimer's Society *Home From Home* report (2007),[31] identified that although people with dementia and care staff benefit greatly from the provision of meaningful activities and recreation, this is very often not provided. Nurses working in care homes have the opportunity to lead in providing stimulating person-centred care that maximises the well-being of those they care for and the work satisfaction for the care staff.

THE WIDER ROLE OF NURSES IN DEMENTIA CARE

The NICE guideline for dementia and Dementia Strategy both provide clear indications of the type and nature of services people with dementia and their carers should expect to have access to. Nurses are recognised as key to leading and implementing quality care provision for people with dementia and the delivery of the national quality standards such as those for dementia.[9]

Health promotion and healthy lifestyle choices are increasingly seen as important in preventing or delaying the onset of dementia and in enabling people who have dementia to maintain their well-being. Across the spectrum of areas in which nurses provide care we all have opportunities to promote healthy living and lifestyle choices and a vital role in reducing the onset and incidence of dementia, as well as supporting people with dementia to maintain well-being through promoting healthy choices in terms of dietary intake, exercise and social activity.

ETHICAL PRACTICE

The person with dementia's life story or 'narrative' enables identification of the person's past life, biography and autobiography and recognition of other important figures in that person's life.[32] This information can be crucial in informing the application of any notions of consent or capacity in the care and treatment of that person. Providing quality information at the right time and identifying the person's 'unique biography' is the basis for good nursing assessment. A partnership model between the person with dementia and the professionals[33] can be placed at the core of nursing roles and interventions for diagnosis, assessment and care planning with people with dementia and their carers.

People with dementia are able to express their views and wishes[34] and the nurse must strive to ensure that this is clearly demonstrated within any process of assessment. Engaging in the assessment of people with dementia, as in all areas of nursing practice, requires a consideration of the ethics of our action or inaction. Do we assume our role gives us a right to ask the person questions about their life?[35] In seeking the person's consent to the process of assessment, the aims and objectives must be clearly stated. Do we always clearly identify why the questions are being asked and what they will be used for? If not, are we acting truthfully and honestly? In completing nursing assessments with someone experiencing dementia, we must be aware of the potential that we are using our position of trust with the person we are assessing to somehow 'trick' them into full disclosure of their experiences, thoughts and plans, without informing them of the potential consequences of this for their future care and treatment.

Acting 'ethically' in any given nursing situation with a person with dementia will require the nurse to pay attention to conflicts of values within herself and between herself and others.[36] In caring for people experiencing dementia, the nurse is frequently faced with the dilemma of balancing the person's 'best interests' with their personhood and right to self determination. Increasingly, as nurses we find it easy to talk of 'recognising the person' not the illness and of promoting independence and offering choice in providing care interventions, but truly achieving this in our practice remains a significant challenge in many areas of dementia nursing care. Service user and carer feedback or structured measures of well-being in dementia (such as dementia care mapping) can enable nurses and the teams in which they work to honestly and critically reflect on the care provided and identify improvements meaningful improvements.

Key points

Nursing input for people with dementia should:
- ➤ demonstrate awareness (through education and training) of the needs of people with dementia
- ➤ promote early diagnosis and provision of information and signposting to local support networks
- ➤ provide person-centred care approaches that promote the person's capacity to make choices
- ➤ ensure psychological or behavioural problems experienced are properly assessed and that pharmacological interventions are not seen as the first option
- ➤ ensure care pathways recognise the specific needs of people with dementia.

REFERENCES

1   Department of Health. *Living Well With Dementia: a national dementia strategy.* London: DoH; 2009.

2   National Institute for Health and Clinical Excellence. *Dementia: supporting people with dementia and their carers in health and social care.* London: NICE; 2006.

3   McKeith I, Fairburn A. Biomedical and clinical perspectives. In: Cantley C (ed). *A Handbook of Dementia Care.* Buckingham: Open University Press; 2001.

4   Royal College of Nursing Institute. *Nursing in Memory Clinics* [resource pack]. London, RCN; 1999.

5   Ryan T, Nolan, M, Reid D, *et al.* Using the senses framework to achieve relationship-centred dementia care services: a case example. *Dementia.* 2008; 7(1): 71–93.

6   Parsons M. Living at home. In: Cantley C (ed). *A Handbook of Dementia Care.* Buckingham: Open University Press; 2001.

7   National Institute for Health and Clinical Excellence. *Delerium: diagnosis, prevention and management: NICE guideline 103.* London: NHICE; 2010. www.nice.org.uk/guidance/CG103

8   *World Alzheimer's Day Bulletin.* London: Alzheimer's Disease International; 2001.

9   National Institute for Health and Clinical Excellence. *Dementia Quality Standards.* London: NICE; 2010.

10 Keady J, Gilliard J. Testing times: the experience of neuropsychological assessment for people with suspected Alzheimer's disease. In: Harris PB (ed). *The Person with Alzheimer's Disease: pathways to understanding the Experience.* Baltimore, MD: John Hopkins University Press; 2002.

11 Moniz-Cook E, Agar S, Gibson G, *et al.* A preliminary study of the effects of early intervention with people with dementia and their families in a memory clinic. *Aging and Mental Health.* 1998; 2(3): 199–211.

12 Stanley D, Cantley C. Assessment care planning and care management. In: Cantley C (ed). *A Handbook of Dementia Care.* Buckingham: Open University Press; 2001.

13 Keady J, Gilliard J. The early experience of Alzheimer's disease: implications for partnership and practice. In: Adams T, Clarke C (eds). *Dementia Care: developing a partnership in practice.* Edinburgh: Churchill Livingstone; 1999.

14 Wilkinson H. *The Perspectives of People with Dementia: research methods and motivation.* London: Jessica Kingsley Publishers, 2002.

15 South West Yorkshire Partnership NHS Foundation Trust. *Dementia Toolkit.* 2008. Available at: www.southwestyorkshire.nhs.uk/documents/832.pdf (accessed May 2011).

16 South West Yorkshire Partnership Foundation Trust. *Portrait of a Life – a multimedia toolkit for life story work.* SWYPFT; 2010.

17 Woods R. Psychological 'therapies' in dementia. In: Woods R (ed). *Psychological Problems of Ageing: assessment, treatment and care.* Chichester: Wiley & Sons Ltd; 1999.

18 Cheston R, Bender M. *Understanding Dementia: the man with the worried eyes.* London: Jessica Kingsley Publishers; 1999.

19 Department of Health. *The Use of Antipsychotic Medication for People with Dementia: time for action.* London: DoH; 2009.

20 SIGN (2006) Scottish Intercollegiate Guidelines Network. *86 Management of Patients with Dementia: a National Clinical Guideline.* Available at: www.sign.ac.uk (accessed May 2011).

21 Marshall M. *State of the Art in Dementia Care*. London: Centre for Policy on Ageing; 1997.

22 Mental Capacity Act 2005. Available at: www.legislation.gov.uk/ukpga/2005/9/ contents (accessed May 2011).

23 Adams T. Kitwood's approach to dementia and dementia care: a critical but appreciative review. *Journal of Advanced Nursing*. 1996; **23**: 948–53.

24 Jenkins D, Price B. Dementia and personhood: a focus for care? *Journal of Advanced Nursing*. 1996; **24**: 84–90.

25 Warren M (cited in Jenkins and Price). On the moral and legal status of abortion. *The Monist*. 1973; **57**(1): 43–61.

26 Alzheimer's Society. *Counting the Cost*. London: Alzheimer's Society; 2009.

27 NHS Confederation. *Acute Awareness: improving hospital care for people with dementia*. London: NHS Confederation; 2010.

28 Mulrooney CP. *Competencies Needed by Formal Care Givers to Enhance Elder Quality of Life: the utility of the 'person and relationship-centred care giving (PRCC) trait'*. Adelaide: 16th Congress of the International Association of Gerontology; 1997.

29 National Mental Health Development Unit. *Let's Respect*. London: NMHDU; 2006. Available at: www.nmhdu.org.uk (accessed May 2011).

30 Tolson D, Smith M, Knight P. An investigation of the components of best nursing practice in the care of acutely ill, hospitalised older patients with coincidental dementia: a multi-method design. *Journal of Advanced Nursing*. 1999; **30**(5): 1127–36.

31 Alzheimer's Society. *Home from Home*. London: Alzheimer's Society; 2007.

32 McCormack B. *The Person of the Voice: narrative identities in informed consent*. Presentation abstract of the *Journal of Dementia Care* Conference, Dublin, 2001.

33 Keady J. *Early Intervention in Dementia: a review of service responses*. Presented to the *Journal of Dementia Care* Conference, Dublin, 2001.

34 Cantley C (ed). *A Handbook of Dementia Care*. Buckingham: Open University Press; 2001.

35 Barker PJ. *Assessment in Psychiatric and Mental Health Nursing: in search of the whole person*. Cheltenham: Stanley Thornes; 1997.

36 Johns C. Framing learning through reflection within Carper's fundamental ways of knowing in nursing. *Journal of Advanced Nursing*. 1995; **22**: 226–34.

CHAPTER 9

Dementia: an occupational therapist's perspective

Mary Duggan

INTRODUCTION

Until recently it has been felt that dementia occupies a shadowy place in public and professional awareness. However, with the publication of the National Dementia Strategy,[1] the needs of people with dementia are becoming better publicised. The core of the strategy is the ambition to enable people to live well with dementia, and it can be argued that occupational therapy has a key role to play in making this possible.

Occupation is a word in common usage that has a highly specific meaning to the occupational therapy profession. Kielhofner[2] defines human occupation as 'doing culturally meaningful work, play or daily living tasks … in the contexts of one's physical and social world'. Occupational therapy is directly concerned with the individual's ability to meet their personal needs for engagement in activity, and the demands placed on them by their social and physical environment. The role of the occupational therapist is to work with individuals whose ability to meet these needs is impaired by illness or disability.

We exist within a complex matrix of social networks, physical environments, occupations and activities. They contribute to the maintenance of our identity. Dementia cannot be fully understood unless it is seen in the context of the individual's physical, social and occupational setting and their experience of it. This chapter explores:

➤ the impact of dementia on engagement in activity
➤ the assessment of occupational performance
➤ occupational therapy interventions.

THE IMPACT OF DEMENTIA ON ENGAGEMENT IN ACTIVITY

The Model of Human Occupation[2] is founded on the belief that meaningful occupation is central to our well-being and that human occupation can best be understood as a dynamic system that involves:

➤ physical and social environments
➤ skills
➤ habituation
➤ personal causation (motivation).

Physical environment

The physical environment tends to become less accessible for us as we age. Decreasing energy and loss of physical fitness makes us less mobile. Places where we like to spend our time or that we need to visit become less easy to get to or to move about in. The physical environment does not just relate to places and spaces. It also involves the materials and tools that we use to perform activities. We select some of these because of their functionality, but many of the objects that we surround ourselves with are chosen as an expression of our personalities.

Dementia may initially produce disorientation in place, making it harder for the individual to make their way about unfamiliar places. In the later stages of dementia, the individual may lose the ability to recognise familiar places (*see* Case Study 9.1) and possessions. The physical environment, far from being a place of security and comfort, may become strange and threatening.

Case Study 9.1

Louise began to turn up at the local police station almost every day. No longer able to recognise her own home, and frightened by finding herself in what seemed to be a strange house, she took the logical course of going to the police. She was confident that they would take her home, which of course they did. It did not take long for the police to realise that she needed help and to refer her to specialist services.

Social environment

We belong to a varied social network: family, friends, colleagues, acquaintances; people who provide the interaction that we enjoy and the services that we need. The process of ageing tends to diminish the social environment through reduced mobility and bereavement.

The impairment of short-term memory experienced in the early stages of dementia may lead to forgetting the names of familiar people. The embarrassment that this produces may make the person with dementia less willing to seek out social contact, beginning a gradual process of social withdrawal. Added to this, it is known that people tend to avoid a person who has been diagnosed with dementia, and one of the first things to change is often the individual's social network. As the dementia progresses, the individual may experience increasing difficulty with memory and with word-finding. The loss of communication skills contributes to difficulty in maintaining social relationships. The person may increasingly withdraw from challenging situations. Family and friends are likely to find communication with the person with dementia becoming more and more frustrating, as their conversation becomes repetitive and focused on past events. In the later stages of dementia, the individual may lose the ability to recognise familiar people, which is in itself a profound form of bereavement. The ability to initiate and maintain social contact becomes progressively reduced.

We primarily experience ourselves as individuals through our interaction with others. Loss of this ability means that it becomes increasingly difficult for the person with dementia to maintain a sense of self, let alone self-worth.

Skills

Occupational behaviour is enabled by a wide range of physical, cognitive and interpersonal skills. Dementia is characterised by a gradual impairment of skills that may manifest in progressively deteriorating memory, loss of attention span, reduced intellectual performance, communication difficulties, loss of judgement and loss of capacity for abstract thought. In the later stages there may also be progressive and significant loss of physical functioning. The loss of skills results in an increasing inability to engage in purposeful occupational behaviour. In addition to this, it is likely that through an honest desire to reduce risk, the carers of the person with dementia deliberately reduce the range of activities that the individual can engage in, thus further eroding their ability to practise and maintain skills.

Habituation

Each of us has a repertoire of life-roles, and this role-set plays a large part in our sense of identity. Often, when meeting someone for the first time, we ask them what they do. Our role-set naturally changes as we move through life, including roles related to family, friends, work, study, community involvement and leisure activity. It tends to reduce as we get older. This loss of roles is linked to factors already mentioned: retirement, increased infirmity, loss of mobility, a reduced social environment. Every role has some value to us, and the loss of a valued role can lead to loss of self-esteem, and contribute to loss of identity.

Our ability to function effectively within our role-set is influenced by the skills that we have, and the behavioural routines that we develop. The loss of skills, described above, sets in train a vicious spiral: the individual becomes less able to engage in roles and their reduced engagement brings with it a corresponding loss of opportunity to use and maintain skills. In addition, the loss of a particular role means a loss of the routines that support it, and therefore loss of some of the structure that enables us to make sense of our lives. Routines are dependent on our ability to remember them, and therefore may be lost as the individual's memory deteriorates. However, encouraging and supporting the person with dementia to maintain their roles and routines may be a major factor in maintaining their skills, engagement and independence.

Motivation

Personal causation is the extent to which we feel more or less competent or skilled at particular activities. Based on our experience of success, it influences our choice of activity or occupation, and produces the drive to engage in activity. It is affected by the values that we place on activities and our personal interests. Any reduction in the opportunity to experience skill, competence and mastery is likely to lead to a loss of motivation to engage in activity.

The loss of skills that is a major feature of dementia will inevitably result in the person with dementia experiencing failure in activities at which they were previously competent or even highly skilled. This contributes to the increasing spiral of withdrawal and disengagement.

The impact of dementia on occupational performance

➤ Dementia impairs the ability of the individual to function within their normal physical and social environment.
➤ Dementia is associated with progressive loss of roles and the routines that sustain them.
➤ Dementia is associated with loss of physical, cognitive and social function.
➤ Dementia is likely to reduce the individual's expectation of competence.
➤ People with dementia are treated differently from others.

ASSESSMENT OF OCCUPATIONAL PERFORMANCE

It is perhaps more important in the assessment of the person with dementia than in any other clinical area that the assessment is genuinely holistic. This involves determining the impact of dementia on all aspects of the individual's life and experience. The contribution of occupational therapy is to assess the impact of dementia on an individual's occupational function and performance, and the Model of Human Occupation[2] (described above) gives a framework for this. The areas that should be assessed include:

➤ the individual's ability to perform required and desired activities within their normal physical and social environment

➤ the extent to which the individual's physical and social environments support or impede their functioning
➤ the roles that the individual wishes or needs to engage in
➤ the ability of the individual to maintain the routines that support these roles
➤ the skills demanded by roles and routines, and the extent to which the individual possesses these skills
➤ the individual's motivation or disposition towards required and desired activities, roles and routines, and their expectation and experience of competence.

There is no universal assessment that covers all of these. However, there is a range of assessment tools and approaches that can provide a comprehensive evaluation of the needs, capabilities and aspirations of the person with dementia. The therapist should not make the assumption that dementia precludes the use of assessments that require verbal response, such as semi-structured interviews. Assessment should combine both observation and interview where possible. Furthermore, any observation of task performance will only be fully meaningful if carried out in the setting in which the individual would normally perform that activity.

Recently, interest in working with people's life stories has been growing and there is increasing evidence of its effectiveness as an intervention with people with dementia. It also has a part to play in the assessment process from an occupational perspective. If we can understand how an individual has come to make occupational choices through their lives, and how this has been influenced by their values, interests and life experiences, we will be better placed to support them in continuing to engage in occupations and activities that are important to them, even when they begin to find it difficult to express choice verbally. A Life Story Network has recently been developed, which is a valuable source of information and ideas.[3]

Occupational Performance History Interview II[4]

Originally developed as a generic measure of occupational performance, this semi-structured interview has been modified to match it more closely to the principles of the Model of Human Occupation. It explores:
➤ the roles that make up an individual's lifestyle
➤ the ways that the individual organises and uses their time
➤ critical life events
➤ the individual's occupational environments, including home, productive activity and leisure, and taking into account the physical and social aspects of those environments
➤ the factors that influence choice of activity
➤ the individual's life story.

The assessment is summarised into three rating scales (each four-point):

➤ the Occupational Identity Scale – the extent to which the individual has goals, values, interests and expectation of success

➤ the Occupational Competence Scale – the extent to which the individual is able to engage satisfactorily in occupational behaviour

➤ the Occupational Behaviour Settings Scale – the extent to which the individual's physical and social environments support their choice of activity, and the extent to which chosen activities match their interests, abilities and personal resources.

Although this assessment seems lengthy on initial inspection, it can be broken down into modules and used over an appropriate period of time. It provides a rich picture of the things that an individual wants and needs to do, and the barriers to effective occupational performance. The authors state that it is suitable for adults who can reflect on and talk about their life history, including people with mild to moderate dementia.

Assessment of Motor and Process Skills[5]

The Assessment of Motor and Process Skills (AMPS) is designed to assess how an individual's motor and process skills affect their ability to carry out activities of daily living (ADL). The assessment is based on the observation of the individual carrying out selected daily living tasks from a specific range. The AMPS allows the individual to choose tasks that are meaningful to them, and can be carried out in any relevant setting.

➤ *Motor skills* – the 'observable, goal directed actions that the person enacts during the performance of ADL tasks to move oneself or the task objects'. Related to posture, mobility, co-ordination and strength.

➤ *Process skills* – the 'observable actions of performance the person enacts to logically sequence the actions of the ADL task performance over time'. Related to attention, concept formation, organisation, planning and ability to adapt.

The tasks are calibrated according to their relative difficulty. In addition, each rater is given a calibration factor to adjust the raw scores in order to eliminate bias arising from rater severity. Recent research[6] indicates that the AMPS is able to distinguish between cognitively well people and people with dementia. The assessment analyses occupational performance and identifies actions that are not carried out effectively.

Pool Activity Level Instrument[7]

The assessments described above enable the therapist to identify the occupations, roles and routines that are important to the individual, and to gauge the extent to which motor and cognitive impairment may reduce or prevent engagement in meaningful activity. The Pool Activity Level Instrument (PAL) closes the loop, as it were, by enabling the identification of the developmental level that a person with dementia is at and suggesting how activity can be structured to support continuing engagement in that activity. Based on an understanding of developmental processes, the PAL checklist uses the following developmental levels.

➤ *Planned activity level* – the individual is able to work towards task completion, but may need assistance with problem solving.

➤ *Exploratory activity level* – the individual can carry out familiar tasks, but is likely to be more interested in the experience of being engaged in activity than in the end result. They may need assistance in sequencing the activity.

➤ *Sensory activity level* – the individual is focused on immediate physical sensation. At this level, people need assistance to perform simple tasks, and these tasks should give the person plenty of opportunity to experience a range of sensations.

➤ *Reflex activity level* – the individual may not be aware of their environment or of physical sensations. Movements that occur are not purposeful, but are in reflex to stimuli. Activities at this level will involve direct sensory stimulation, introducing a single sensation at a time.

The PAL Action Plan enables the therapist to identify activities that the individual is likely to be motivated to take part in, and describes in some detail how to structure that activity to maximise its effectiveness. The PAL is a highly effective tool for multidisciplinary care planning – it enables staff and carers to structure all of the activities that the person with dementia takes part in to ensure that engagement is maintained and that activity is meaningful and a positive experience.

Assessment of risk

There is great concern, rightly so, with the assessment of risk. Thom and Blair[8] describe the role of occupational therapy in identifying actual risks to the individual through the use of functional assessment based on observation and interview. They stress the importance of fully engaging with both patient and carers in this process. They acknowledge the tension that is present between risk prevention and the rights of the individual to take risks, and argue for a balance between risk and quality of life (*see* Case Studies 9.2 and 9.3). A useful and comprehensive guidance document has recently been issued by the Department of Health.[8]

Of course, it is vital to be aware of the risks, and to carry out an assessment of the potential and actual impact of those risks on the individual. Thom and Blair suggest, based on the literature reviewed, that the following areas should be considered:[9]

Case Study 9.2

Annie was admitted to hospital because of concerns about her leaving her house and 'wandering'. In casual conversation, she began to reminisce about her earlier life, especially during World War Two. She had always loved boats and sailing. She was one of the people that risked their lives piloting small craft across the Channel to evacuate soldiers from the Dunkirk beaches. Now, some 50 years on, she was faced with the prospect of not being allowed to take any risks at all. This conversation caused the whole team to re-evaluate their attitudes towards Annie and risk, and certainly gave a completely different sense of proportion.

Case Study 9.3

Adam had been admitted to hospital because he was a high suicide risk. He knew that he had dementia, and hated the thought of living with it. He also desperately wanted to go home. The team worked very carefully with Adam and his family, and came to the agreement that, while there would be a risk of him harming or even killing himself, this was outweighed by his wish to be at home. The care plan that supported his discharge from hospital provided daily supportive contact that enabled the team to monitor his mood closely and sensitively. He was able to remain in his own home for a further 18 months before having to move into long-term care.

➤ physical risks – cuts, falls, impaired mobility
➤ ability to operate household appliances safely
➤ personal risks – self-care, nutrition, medication compliance, continence, dressing
➤ coping with the outdoor environment – getting lost, going out at night, driving, shopping
➤ general risks – financial management, risk of being abused, home security, dealing with emergencies, communication ability, smoking, alcohol abuse.

In addition to risks of accidental self-harm described above, the risk of deliberate self-harm should not be ignored. In the earlier stages of dementia, the individual may well have insight into their illness. As with any progressive and indeed terminal illness, the individual is likely to question whether or not they wish to continue to live. Thoughts of suicide would not be unusual, and may be acted on.

INTERVENTION

There is an argument that occupational therapists who work with people with dementia tend to focus their energies on functional assessment, and specifically on risk management. In a discussion of the role of the occupational therapist in continuing care settings, Perrin describes 'the craft of the occupational therapist, who must impose order upon the chaos of pain, disruption and dysfunction by the artful manipulation of occupations'.[10] It is vital that the occupational therapist not only identifies the barriers to occupational performance, as described above, but also uses a range of interventions to enable the individual with dementia to continue to engage in meaningful and purposeful activity, and to live as independently as possible in the least restrictive environment compatible with agreed levels of safety. The interventions used traditionally involve:

➤ modification of the physical environment
➤ modification of the social environment
➤ the use, modification or adaptation of purposeful activities or occupations.

Dementia is a progressive condition, and therapeutic intervention may move along a continuum from rehabilitation or re-ablement to adaptation and compensation with an overarching focus on maintaining engagement and personhood. Perrin and May[11] argue that the traditional rehabilitative approach, which has an ultimate goal of withdrawing support and increasing independence, is ineffective in the context of dementia care. They suggest that an understanding of the interrelationship of occupation and well-being is of central importance, and that a 'state of "wellness", rather than of "health" is a more appropriate goal'.

Environmental modification

It is important that the individual's physical environment supports them in carrying out the activities that they need and want to do. The most significant environment is the individual's home and its surroundings. The therapist has a responsibility to guide the individual and their carers in eliminating unnecessary risk from that environment, but equally has a responsibility to ensure that the home remains a place where the individual can take part in meaningful and valued activity (*see* Case Study 9.4).

Over recent years, there has been an upsurge in the availability of technology that can assist individuals to maintain their independence. A recent study[12] carried out by occupational therapists in Leeds shows how one system can be used to map a person's pattern of activity over the 24-hour period. The Just Checking system enables professionals and carers to plan and monitor care packages for people who live alone, even when they are not able to accurately describe their activity patterns themselves. Staff using the system find that

---

Case Study 9.4

Mary was in the early stages of the dementia process. The AMPS enabled her therapist to look at the coping strategies that she was already using, and to tap into them. Mary kept her washing machine in the garage, and would often put clothes in but then forget about them. The AMPS indicated that she used visual cues to remind her of tasks. Her therapist suggested that each time she put clothes in to wash she left the box of soap powder out on the kitchen counter. This reminded her that she needed to go back and put the clothes in the dryer. This was a much more meaningful and effective coping strategy for Mary than a written list would have been.

---

people with dementia are often better able to cope than had been expected, and a more comprehensive picture of a person's strengths can be established. Furthermore, the system makes it easier to schedule support exactly when it is needed and increases the likelihood of enabling the person to stay in their own home. Telecare now provides a range of devices, such as property exit sensors, fall sensors, flood detectors and pager systems, to monitor specific areas of risk remotely and mobilise assistance if and when needed.

Modifying the social environment is, perhaps, less obvious. The person with dementia may have become increasingly socially isolated. If this is due to lack of confidence in leaving the house, or loss of the ability to make their way to social venues, they may simply need assistance with transport. If they are finding it difficult to engage in activities, the therapist may need to consider introducing them to environments where these activities can be structured to support participation. The current national pilot schemes to develop peer support networks for people with dementia and their carers could point the way for ensuring that there are opportunities for people to maintain participation in activity within their own communities. A recent directory of good practice in Yorkshire and the Humber describes several such schemes.[13]

Perhaps the most significant aspect of modifying the social environment is the work that may need to be carried out with the person's carers. Post-diagnosis education and counselling is extremely important, but the role of carer as expert also needs to be nurtured. Wherever possible, carers should be fully participant in the assessment and care-planning process, so that everyone involved has a shared and clear picture of the person's ability as well as disability, and their hopes and aspirations for the future. The therapist can then explore the ways in which carers can continue to encourage and support the person to live well with dementia (*see* Case Study 9.5).

Case Study 9.5

Janet developed Korsakoff's syndrome while still in her mid-40s. She was admitted to hospital in an acutely confused state: she was confabulating, she had difficulty distinguishing between her dreams and waking experiences and she was frightened about being in hospital. The Occupational Performance History Interview assessment (see above) showed that productive activity was of great significance to her. She had given up a very responsible career because of the increasing deterioration of memory and cognitive functioning that she was experiencing, and was no longer engaging in any activity that was relevant to her and her needs. With encouragement, she chose to cook a meal, something that she would do on her return home. Her therapist used this to establish rapport and also to give Janet a much needed experience of success. Janet began to show rapid improvement. The therapist worked with the team and Janet's family to help her to establish a more meaningful and satisfying routine. Her partner ran a small business, and agreed to give Janet some simple clerical tasks to do. She needed step-by-step instruction and a huge amount of support from him, but this enabled her to re-establish a valued routine. She became happy and confident. She stopped drinking, and knew what coping strategies to use to avoid re-admission.

Activity modification

The core tenet of occupational therapy is that meaningful activity is central to our well-being. Perrin,[14] in a study using the dementia care mapping instrument developed at the University of Bradford by Kitwood, Bredin and others, identified that older people with dementia who are in long-term care spend much of their time unoccupied. There is a strong argument that the failure to provide opportunity for activity, whether this is in the context of a residential care setting or the person's own home, constitutes a form of abuse of people with dementia.[15]

Case Study 9.6

Adam was an active man in his mid-50s when he began to show signs of cognitive impairment. He still retained a degree of insight, and found it difficult to come to terms with the prospect of a progressive illness. This led to his hospitalisation as a suicide risk. On the ward, he showed a range of behavioural problems. The OPHI-II showed that routine was deeply significant. He had spent many years in the armed forces and still had a very rigid daily structure. He talked with great pride about

---

his past achievements; he had been a skilled leader and was highly respected. He was very clear about what he wanted: to return home, to be able to go for walks, to make himself drinks and snacks. In the ward setting, his own rigid personal routines clashed with the ward routines, leading to Adam expressing his frustration through 'difficult' behaviour. The therapist designed Adam's care plan around his routines, accompanying him on walks and encouraging him to make drinks for himself in his own room. These routines enabled the team to establish a package of support at home that was highly successful. Again, all of the interventions were timed to fit in precisely with his routine, and focused on checking that he was still maintaining his routine safely and successfully. Eventually, Adam needed to go into long-term care. The team helped him to make a smooth transition by finding a home that was able to create a care programme around his routines and activities. He still goes out with a member of staff for a daily run.

Therapists working with people in the early stages of dementia are likely to focus their energies on maintaining routines, skills, and the individual's participation in activities and occupations of their choice (*see* Case Study 9.6). In the later stages of dementia, especially where the individual is functioning at the reflex or sensory levels described in the PAL tool, the meaningfulness of an activity may not always be apparent to the therapist (*see* Case Study 9.7). Careful observation and dialogue with carers may help the therapist to make an activity more meaningful and satisfying.

Case Study 9.7

Freddie began the multi-sensory session by crawling about on the floor. He often did this on the ward. He was giving the impression of being very busy and concentrating hard on what he was doing. The therapy assistant suggested that he might be sweeping up. She gave him a brush, and he proceeded to sweep the entire floor, with great satisfaction. Here, the therapy assistant helped him to engage in an overtly purposeful activity. Sometimes, Freddie liked to stand at the old-fashioned wash-tub. He needed two people to help him to maintain his balance. He would enjoy pushing and pulling the scrubbing board back and forth. While there was no apparent external meaning to this activity, Freddie would focus on it for long periods of time. He was working. In fact, the only way to persuade him to rest was to suggest that it was time for a tea break. In this instance, it did not matter that the therapist did not understand the meaning of the activity; Freddie did.

There may also be an argument that when working with people in the later stages of dementia, where the focus of activity is on stimulating the senses and maintaining social contact, the nature of the activity also becomes important for staff and carers. Working with an individual who can give minimal feedback is tiring. Here, it is vital to have a wide range of activities that can be engaged in for as long as the individual's attention span allows, and that avoids monotony for all concerned. The occupational therapist can play a vital role here in suggesting suitable activities, and also showing how to structure or modify them to enable the individual to engage. The concept that Perrin and May[11] describe as the 'bubble' can inform practice. This bubble is the boundary beyond which the person with dementia cannot perceive their surroundings. The bubble shrinks progressively. In this phase, the work of the therapist is one of reaching out, making and maintaining contact, through whichever activity and medium works in that moment. The goal of occupational therapy, and indeed of the multi-professional team working with people with dementia, is ultimately to maintain the individual's sense of self and, most importantly, their sense of being a valued person.

Key points

➤ Dementia impairs the ability of the individual to engage in meaningful occupation.

➤ Occupational therapy assessment of the person with dementia should encompass their ability to perform the activities required by their roles and environment, the extent to which their physical and social environment supports their engagement in activity and their motivation towards activities and occupations.

➤ Assessment should draw on a range of approaches, including the use of standardised assessments, observation and interview. Therapists should strive for balance between the management of risk and the rights of the individual to take risks.

➤ Therapeutic interventions with the individual with dementia may involve:
  – modifying the physical environment so that it supports engagement in occupation
  – modifying the social environment so that it supports engagement in occupation
  – modifying or adapting purposeful activities or occupations to support engagement.

➤ The overall focus of assessment and therapeutic intervention with the person with dementia should be to maintain their engagement and sense of self.

ACKNOWLEDGEMENTS

I am grateful to Katie Barker for the Case Studies, and to Jane Currie, General Manager and James Waplington, Clinical Manager (both at Older People's Services, South West Yorkshire Mental Health Trust, Wakefield, UK) for their support.

REFERENCES

1　Department of Health. *Living Well with Dementia: a national dementia strategy.* London: DoH; 2009.

2　Kielhofner G. *A Model of Human Occupation: theory and application.* 2nd ed. Baltimore, MD: Williams & Wilkins; 1995.

3　Life Story Network. www.lifestorynetwork.org.uk (accessed May 2011).

4　Kielhofner, G, Mallinson T, Crawford C, *et al. Occupational Performance History Interview II. Model of Human Occupation Clearing House.* www.uic.edu/moho/assess/ophi%202.html (accessed May 2011).

5　Fisher AG. *Assessment of Motor and Process Skills.* 3rd ed. Fort Collins, CO: Three Star Press; 1999.

6　Robinson SE, Fisher AG. Functional and cognitive differences between cognitively-well people and people with dementia. *British Journal of Occupational Therapy.* 1999; 62(10): 466–71.

7　Pool J. *The Pool Activity Level (PAL) Instrument.* London: Jessica Kingsley Publishers; 1999.

8　Manthorp J, Moriarty J. *Nothing Ventured, Nothing Gained: risk guidance for people with dementia.* London: Social Care Workforce Research Unit, King's College, for the Department of Health; 2010. Available at: www.dh.gov.uk/dr_consum_dh/groups/dh_digitalassets/@dh/@eh/@ps/documents/digitalasset/dh_121493.pdf (accessed August 2011).

9　Thom KM, Blair SEC. Risk in dementia – assessment and management: a literature review. *British Journal of Occupational Therapy.* 1998; 61(10): 441–7.

10　Perrin T. Don't despise the fluffy bunny: a reflection from practice. *British Journal of Occupational Therapy.* 2001; 64(3): 129–34.

11　Perrin T, May H. *Wellbeing in Dementia: an occupational approach for therapists and carers.* London: Churchill Livingstone; 2000.

12　Roworth Gaunt C, Ridout A, Wormald G, *et al. Just Checking Telecare 1 Year Report: Giving people with dementia a voice.* Leeds Partnership NHS Foundation Trust and Just Checking; 2009. Available at: www.justchecking.co.uk/downloads/pdfs/leeds_report.pdf (accessed May 2011).

13　Yorkshire and Humber Improvement Partnership. *Inspiring Innovation in Dementia: Regional Directory 2010.* YHIP, Department of Health; 2010. Available at: www.yhip.org.uk/silo/files/yhip-dementia-innovation-directory.pdf (accessed May 2011).

14　Perrin T. Occupational need in severe dementia: a descriptive study. *Journal of Advanced Nursing.* 1999; 25(5): 934–41.

15　Marshall MJ, Hutchinson, SA. A critique of the use of activities with persons with Alzheimer's disease: a systematic literature review. *Journal of Advanced Nursing.* 2001; 35(4): 488–96.

CHAPTER 10

Social aspects of the assessment and treatment of dementia

Dorrie Ball and Nick Farrar

THE DEMENTIA 'EPIDEMIC'

On 21 September 2009, World Alzheimer's Day, a report published by Alzheimer's Disease International presented global figures indicating the predicted dementia 'epidemic'. In 2010 an estimated 35.6 million people worldwide will be living with dementia; by 2030 this figure is estimated to reach 65.7 million; and by 2050 a further increase to 115.4 million is estimated.[1] Much of this predicted increase is thought to be due to increasing numbers of older people in low- and middle-income countries. Associated problems related to this growth are likely to be lack of awareness, under-diagnosis and stigma caused by such developments. Some three years earlier a report, commissioned by the 15 Asia Pacific members of Alzheimer's Disease International, concluded that the number of people with dementia in that region would rise from 14 million currently to 65 million by 2050 and that the number of new cases will increase from 4 million to 20 million over the same period.[2] There is, however, a disparity within the region, more information being available within the more developed countries than many developing countries, the latter having 'limited awareness of dementia; an assumption that dementia is a natural part of ageing; and inadequate human and financial resources to meet care needs' (Statistics[2]).

In the UK there are currently about 700 000 people with a form of dementia, representing one in 14 people over 65 years of age and one in six over 80 years of age. By 2021 there will be an estimated increase to 940 000 and by 2051 this figure will reach 1.7 million.[3] Recent research by the Alzheimer's Society has shown that even within the UK there is a very surprising lack of dementia awareness, results indicating that only half of the population realise there is no cure for dementia, approximately a third mistakenly agreeing that dementia was a 'natural part of ageing' and a quarter believing there was no way to reduce risk.[4]

The term dementia defines a group of syndromes characterised by progressive decline in cognition, caused by disease or trauma, and usually associated with increasing age. There are many sub-types, but the most prevalent is Alzheimer's disease, accounting for approximately 70% of cases, followed by vascular dementia, accounting for 10–20% of cases.[5] Incidence of dementia rises rapidly with age (i.e. the rate of occurrence of new cases during a specific time period). Early onset dementia (between 40 and 50 years of age) is uncommon and usually linked to specific risk factors such as Down's syndrome, whereas prevalence studies indicate that dementia doubles approximately every five years after the age of 65.[5] However, whilst ageing appears to be the greatest risk factor in developing dementia, it must be stressed that dementia is not part of the normal ageing process.

PERSPECTIVES ON WORKING WITH OLDER PEOPLE IN THE UK

In order to discuss the social aspects of the assessment and treatment of dementia, this chapter will explore the social context of older people, from theoretical and professional perspectives, with particular emphasis on the changes which have taken place in the last two decades, so that issues of intervention and potential options in addressing dementia from a social perspective can be located in a current and realistic context. Other important issues to be considered include legislative and policy influences that have changed the role of social workers and other professionals, and placed increasing emphasis on the need for multidisciplinary working and the involvement of users and carers in the assessment process and the ongoing care.

It has been suggested that working with older people in social care settings has in the past tended to be seen as routine and undemanding, requiring little expertise or training – a notion that is strongly challenged as a negative view, reflecting society's ageist and discriminatory attitude to older people.[6] This attitude may be manifested in a number of ways, such as direct oppression (e.g. abuse in its many forms) or more subtle forms, such as derogatory or patronising language, stereotypical humour in media presentations or jokes, or infantilisation – a process which sadly has often been observed in residential or other forms of institution (scheduled 'toileting' times, use of first names, etc.). A further significant element of this view of older people is the tendency to see ageing predominantly in medical terms, and the ageing process as a period of degeneration rather than development, with inevitable links to illness and infirmity – the 'what do you expect at your age?' syndrome. More recent comments have claimed that 'ageism' is manifest in health and social care, in areas such as: government policies; the organisation and staffing of services for older people; the differential development of procedures for children and adults; and the language used to describe older people.[7] John Bond and colleagues have suggested there are a number of theoretical approaches to the study of ageing, emanating from biological, psychological and sociological perspectives, which focus on different aspects of the ageing process.[8] These approaches are not right or wrong, simply different – and therefore resulting in different interventions. Similarly, in the wealth of literature emerging in relation to dementia, there are seen to be different disciplines, with different conceptual frameworks, which result in different ways of studying and interpreting the same phenomenon. However, these approaches are not necessarily contradictory but may be complementary, each making a contribution to the understanding of dementia. Thus they could be seen as contributing to a 'holistic' approach, a framework which is increasingly demanded by current policies and practice, such as multidisciplinary assessment.

In order to work with older people in an anti-oppressive and anti-discriminatory manner, it is essential to regard each older person as an individual, with their own biography, which may be influenced by gender, race/ethnicity, class, sexual orientation, etc. It is also important to encompass changing life expectations over time, for example, potential choices about retirement age, access to travel/holidays, lifelong learning. Developments such as these may in time influence and change attitudes to older people, along with policy directives such as the National Service Framework for Older People, which set national standards and defined service models for the care of older people, the first standard attempting to eliminate discrimination against older people in the provision of services.[9] Whilst this National Service Framework addressed a broad range of policy and service issues, it also had a number of specific points which have significance for dementia care.

Many of the policy developments over the last 10 years since the National Service Framework reflect a growing change in the way we might see older age: *Link Age*[10] set out proposals for a Third Age Service to enable staff from the Department for Work and Pensions and local authorities to set up joint teams of staff. *Opportunity Age*[11] described the government's key strategy for an ageing society. It focused on three key areas: firstly, work and income – achieving greater flexibility for over 50s in continuing careers, managing health conditions and combining work with family (and other) commitments; secondly, active ageing – enabling older people to play a full and active role in society; and, finally, services – that allow people to keep independence and control over their lives as they grow older, even if constrained by the health problems.

Building a Society for all Ages proposed measures 'to help instil a major cultural shift and help Britain prepare for demographic change which is seeing people live longer lives'.[12]

This involved providing support to people to look forward and plan earlier for their longer lives, and making sure that services were suitable when the time comes to use them. It also outlined a number of new measures, including bringing forward a review of the default retirement age and promoting flexible opportunities for 50+ self-employment.

DEVELOPMENTS IN WAYS OF WORKING WITH DEMENTIA

The above theoretical explanations and changing perceptions of ageing have been reflected in the development of approaches to dementia over the last two decades. A leading exponent of new ideas in this field has been Tom Kitwood, whose personal experiences led to a growing interest and later a professional involvement in exploring ways of understanding and working with dementia.[13] Kitwood's ideas presented, initially rather tentatively, a challenge to the medical model that framed dementia as an 'organic mental disorder' or what he termed the 'standard paradigm'. His deepening involvement in enhancing the well-being and quality of care for dementia sufferers placed emphasis on authentic contact and communication, with a focus on 'person-centred care' and supporting family carers. A new method for evaluating the quality of care in formal settings was developed, termed Dementia Care Mapping, which attempted to recognise the standpoint of the person with dementia, with consequent capacity to improve the caring process for both service-users and carers.

Kitwood was not alone in promoting challenges to the bio-medical theories of understanding dementia and the last decade has seen a proliferation of texts developing new approaches to care for people with dementia. It must, however, be pointed out that these innovative approaches have developed in a social and economic climate where there has been a major concern not only about the increasing number of people diagnosed as having dementia, but also about the numbers of older people *per se*, whose increasing health and social care needs are perceived to be a 'burden' on welfare resources.

Many of the recent approaches have expanded on Kitwood's ideas of personhood and communication in dementia care, but there has also been a focus on the quality of care settings and the care environment, the development of a wide range of approaches to practice in this field, an emphasis on working with informal carers and the changes which new policies have effected in this field.[14] A former colleague of Kitwood has attempted to clarify the concept of 'person-centred care' by proposing the VIPS model, which presented four key elements:

V Valuing people with dementia and those who care for them
I treating people as Individuals
P viewing through the Perspective of the person with dementia and
S a positive Social environment to encourage well-being.[15]

A decade on from Kitwood's untimely death, a critical commentary has sum-marised and problematised his contribution to the field of dementia care.[16] Whilst acknowledging his leadership in the extensive development of new con-cepts of dementia and provision of care services, this critique has examined the strengths and also pointed to the limitations and ambiguities of Kitwood's work.

Further research has taken a social science perspective to critically examine the main approaches – bio-medical, social-psychological and socio-geronto-logical – to the study of dementia, to argue for a move away from the focus on the individual to an emphasis on the social, cultural and economic con-text of dementia, which it is claimed provides a needed broader theoretical framework for addressing this area of study.[17] Others, however, have drawn on evidence-based practice from the UK and Europe to claim that psycho-social interventions provided in the early stages of diagnosed dementia can make a valuable contribution to quality of life.[18] This approach takes into account vari-ous aspects of a person's life to identify the type of support that can prevent dis-tress and enhance well-being at this crucial time. This might involve a variety of interventions and services, such as support groups, art therapies, carer support or assistive technologies in the home.

One recent approach to treating dementia, which has attracted considerable attention, was developed by a care-giver and documented by her psycholo-gist son-in-law.[19] Named SPECAL (Specialised Early Care for Alzheimer's), this method emphasises the belief that feelings are more important than facts to the person with dementia. 'When a well-meaning carer points out to the per-son that they have forgotten something … they feel embarrassed and agitated … their over-whelming feeling is that they are not in control.'[20] SPECAL has three basic rules: don't ask the person with dementia questions; never con-tradict them; learn to love their repetitiveness; The aim of these is to retain a sense of well-being and contentment in the person with dementia.[19] Therapeu-tic approaches such as this have, however, contributed to lively debates about whether it is ever ethically acceptable to lie to people with dementia.[21]

A further recent exciting development, which builds on the theme of per-son-centred care, is a workbook which uses a wealth of exercises and activities aimed at connecting with the person with dementia and empowering both them and their carers, in order to achieve good practice and the best care pos-sible.[22]

Perhaps the most impressive collection of research into dementia is an edited collection which draws on the extensive knowledge of researchers, practitioners and professionals as well as the experiences of users of services.[23] Encompassing a very wide range of perspectives, this publication is informed by respect for people with dementia, a commitment to their inclusion in the decision-making processes, support for those giving care and strategies for creating positive changes in practice. One important matter considered is the importance of assessment in relation to people with dementia, and the need for good planning, skills and empathy to achieve best practice in this area.[24]

A recent statutory change which is having impact on the social assessment process in England is the implementation of the Mental Capacity Act 2005, which requires that the wishes of the person being assessed must be taken into account, unless it can be proved that they do not have the capacity to make decisions for themselves. Debates surrounding this complex issue have also focused on the challenges and contradictions imposed by the interface between decision-making processes and the concept of personhood, which offers a holistic approach to the treatment of the person with dementia.[25]

As well as involvement in the assessment process, it is suggested that there are a number of occasions when social workers may encounter people with dementia, which connect medical events (the time of diagnosis, or admission to hospital) with life events, such as loss of particular memory skills, or times when carers cannot cope and respite care is necessary.[26] These require elements of good practice such as the need for continuity of care and the need to support carers and be sensitive to carer stress. Especially important are specialist training, flexibility, accessible information and services and the need for multi-disciplinary teams that include other professionals (p. 152ff).[26] To deliver all of these very important practice developments, investment is needed.

DEVELOPMENTS IN POLICY RELATING TO THE CARE OF OLDER PEOPLE OVER THE LAST TWO DECADES

Community care has a long history, but arguably the most dramatic changes in this country have come about over the last 20 years, driven partly by the need to contain care costs of a population with a rising number of older people.

The NHS and Community Care Act 1990, which introduced the concept of Care Management, ushered in a period of intense government activity, which continues in reshaping the delivery of social and health care. One major focus has been involving users and carers in planning and providing services to attempt to make the system 'a seamless service'. Another has been the separation of assessment of need from provision of services to meet that need, providing a 'gate-keeping' process of resources, as well as targeting those who have the greatest need. Yet another focus has been joint planning and joint target setting.[27] Together these changes have formed part of an ongoing attempt to drive health and social care provision together, whilst keeping the essential differences between health and social care intact – healthcare being free at the point of delivery whilst there is a charge for social care.

Policy developments have included Fair Access to Care Services (FACS),[28] which provided councils with an eligibility framework for delivery of adult social care services in each local area – i.e. who will get a service, and who will not, based on a national set of needs-based criteria. In 2008 the Commission for Social Care Inspection (SCIE) reviewed these criteria and found that the system for assessing eligibility was flawed. It recommended that everyone should have an assessment of their support needs, including information and advice to help them make the right choices, and introduced new eligibility criteria which relate to the urgency of a person's situation.[29] These proposals have been developed as part of the government's current 'personalisation' agenda – popularly known as *Putting People First.*[30] This ministerial concordat established formal collaboration between central and local government, the sector's professional leadership, providers and the regulator. It set out shared aims and values, and stated that the sector would work across agendas with users and carers to transform people's experience of local support and services, to ensure that older people, people with chronic conditions, disabled people and people with mental health problems should have the best possible quality of life and the equality of independent living. This included the need to work for people with dementia as well as those without cognitive impairment.

It could be argued that the many sequelae to *Putting People First* are in essence a retread of Care Management created by the NHS and Community Care Act 1990, but with the added emphasis of more preventative services, giving service users apparently more control over their care. *Shaping the Future of Care Together*[31] is the most recent government green paper which attempts to create a national debate about the future of paying for adult social care, an area of concern in the current economic climate and the demographic pressures in the UK. All these policies have had, and continue to have, significant implications for professionals and users alike. With their focus on user involvement and setting national standards and targets, they may help professionals deliver more appropriate services. Getting the balance right is one of the biggest challenges to be faced in this environment. Working out how to pay for care and the balance between the individual and the state is crucial. Risk as an essential part of health and social care has also been driven up the agenda for many reasons over the last 10 years. What we must be aware of is that risk-awareness does not become part of our plans to the detriment of appropriate risk-taking.

DEVELOPMENTS IN POLICY RELATING TO DEMENTIA OVER THE LAST DECADE

There has been a steady stream of policy developments relating to dementia over the last 10 years. In 2000 the Audit Commission published its *Forget Me Not* report.[32] Key findings included: only one-half of GPs believed it important to look actively for signs of dementia and to make an early diagnosis, and less than one-half of GPs felt that they had received sufficient training. There was a lack of clear information, counselling, advocacy and support for people with dementia and their family carers, and there was insufficient supply of specialist home care. The Audit Commission found little improvement when reviewing change two years later.[33]

The National Institute for Health and Clinical Excellence (NICE) and the SCIE published a joint Clinical Guideline on the management of dementia in 2006.[34] Key recommendations included: integrated working across all agencies; provision of memory assessment services as a point of referral for diagnosis of dementia; assessment, support and treatment (where needed) for carers; assessment and treatment of non-cognitive symptoms and behaviour that challenges; dementia-care training for all staff working with older people; and improvement of care for people with dementia in general hospitals.

In February 2007, the Alzheimer's Society published *Dementia UK*.[35] Its recommendations included making dementia an explicit national health and social care priority and the need to improve the quality of services provided for people with dementia and their carers.

The National Audit Office published the findings of its review of dementia services, *Improving Services and Support for People with Dementia*, in July 2007.[36] This report was critical about the quality of care received by people with dementia and their families. It found that the size and availability of specialist community mental health teams was extremely variable, and that confidence of GPs in spotting the symptoms of dementia was poor and lower than it had been in 2000. It also commented on deficiencies in carer support. The report concluded that overall services are not currently delivering value for money to taxpayers or people with dementia and their families.

The Department of Health's *End of Life Strategy* was published in July 2008.[37] End-of-life care for people with dementia is an underdeveloped area which required specific attention.

The National Dementia Strategy was published in early 2009.[38] It dealt with three key themes: better knowledge and the removal of stigma; good and early diagnosis; and a proper range of services. The detail of the strategy is too long to replicate here; however, supported by a delivery plan and a commissioning plan, the whole approach was based on clear and invaluable user and carer involvement, which augurs well for its vision of future services. It remains to be seen how well the steps outlined will be funded.

WHAT DOES THIS MEAN FOR PEOPLE WITH DEMENTIA?

The *Forget Me Not* report[32] and its review revealed that despite the changes so far made, where one lives still dictates the quality of care one receives and structural changes cannot deliver changes of themselves. Many of the policy developments since then have attempted to address these issues and the new

Dementia Strategy is a massive step forward. Critics have suggested that the strategy did not cover the issue of people with dementia being given antipsychotic medication and did not sufficiently support more research. However, both of these criticisms have been swiftly addressed. Questions as to resourcing new and better services can always be raised, and we should be wary of complacency. Much will depend on professional attitudes to these changes as to whether they have a significant impact on the way in which people are cared for. What we can say is that the stated intention is to change things for the better, and that the potential for more integrated assessment and provision of care is there.

THE ROLE OF CARERS

There have been several legislative and policy developments in recent years which have relevance for carers of people with dementia. The Carers (Recognition and Services) Act 1995 was the first piece of legislation to formally recognise the role of carers. It ushered in the right of carers, who were providing substantial amounts of care on a regular basis, to have a separate assessment of their needs and ability to care, which local authorities were required to take into account when making decisions about providing services. Subsequent research findings[39] suggested that care managers' insight and understanding of the legislation was limited, there was a lack of clear policy at local level and little specific training in relation to roles and responsibilities towards carers. Additionally, carers' knowledge of their rights to assessment was limited.

Recognition of some of these limitations had led to the National Carers Project in 1998, which resulted in the Carers' National Strategy.[40] This strategy placed emphasis on providing support to carers at key points in the caring process, and helping in the development of relevant skills. An important element of the strategy was the notion of enabling carers the choice as to whether to care or not. However, achieving these apparently positive aims may not have been realistic, as most agencies tend to see carers as a resource, and therefore attempt to maintain them in their role as far as possible.[41]

Subsequent legislation in the form of the Carers and Disabled Children Act 2000 and the Carers (Equal Opportunities) Act 2004 further developed the rights described in the 1995 Act, by giving local authorities power to provide services directly to carers, even if the cared-for person did not wish for an assessment, and helping to ensure that carers are not placed at a disadvantage because of the care they provide.

The government also provided some additional money for carers as part of its modernisation initiative. A specific grant to social services departments – the carers' grant – was introduced in 1999, with a focus on stimulating diversity and flexibility in provision of breaks for carers and/or direct services to support them in the caring role. It has increased annually and has risen to £240 million in 2009/10, with a further rise to £256 million in 2010/11.[42] The amount of the grant in comparison with the actual costs of informal care is small. Past attempts to quantify the costs of informal care have met with difficulties, as the relationship between measuring costs and key aspects of informal care is extremely complex, involving factors such as stress on carers, predictors of breakdown of caring networks and the effects of service interventions.[43] However, it can be assumed that if carers were to withdraw their support, the cost to the state would be colossal. A further point of relevance is that many people in relationships providing caring functions do not describe themselves as 'carers', rather regarding this as part of the close relationship or familial duty, which may particularly be the case with older carers or spouses. Additionally, it has been suggested that there is a pervasive assumption that women possess 'natural caring capacities' and will be available to care. As the largest proportion of informal (and formal) carers are women, caring predominantly for older women, this may reflect negatively on the perception of care arrangements for older people by compounding the negative stereotypes previously referred to.[44]

A national focus on supporting carers is of itself sensible, and necessary. However, studies show that caring for someone with dementia has particular challenges and stresses. Heron[45] has suggested that carers of people with mental health problems have, even prior to current trends, traditionally been seen as a separate group of carers, with a distinct identity. Whilst carers in this group may benefit from generic support, specific needs may include information about the nature and progression of the illness, access to emergency services or short-term intensive interventions in the event of crises. As the profile of dementia has been raised, so has the often hidden experiences of care-givers begun to receive more attention, as shown in the powerful stories presented by 30 carers from different backgrounds, whose personal experiences illustrate a rollercoaster of distress and tragedy, but also inspiration and resilience.[46]

Objective 7 of the 2009 Dementia Strategy stressed that carers are the most important resource available for people with dementia, and it is vital that their right to an assessment is recognised and that there should be an agreed plan to support the important role they play in the care of the person with dementia. Additionally, Objective 3 claims that good-quality information about the illness and the services should be available for people with dementia and their carers.

THE IMPLICATIONS FOR INTERVENTIONS IN THE SOCIAL ASPECTS OF DEMENTIA CARE

We have seen that there is now a much wider range of accepted views on dementia than there was 10 or 15 years ago, which gives us some basis for a more positive view on what can be achieved. The models of 'personhood' and the work on communication with people with dementia show what is possible, along with other new understanding about environment, illness, the person and their interaction with carers. We know that people with dementia can have valued lives, and that there is much that can be done to support this. However, we can see from the Audit Commission analysis in 2000[32] and the National Audit Office review in 2007[36] that there is much variation in services across the country. In relation to the challenges to social care professionals, key elements include a holistic approach to assessment, multidisciplinary teamwork (incorporating the movements towards merging health and social care introduced by many of the government's policies), the development of service provision which addresses equality strategies and issues of partnership, participation and empowerment, which infiltrate all of the above processes.

In relation to people with dementia, assessment and service provision would normally take place within the context of a multidisciplinary community mental health team. The advantages of this service context are that service users and carers receive a dedicated service, rationalised and co-ordinated service provision and specialised professional staff. The disadvantages (as in any multidisciplinary team) are that different professional and organisational cultures, interests and priorities can impede the assessment and service delivery process.[47] The challenge within this scenario is to achieve a balance between the social and medical models of dementia care.

A core theme of the assessment and care planning process is the emphasis on a needs-led approach – identifying individual needs and attempting to meet these needs – rather than slotting people into existing resources, and this is central to the 'personalisation' agenda influencing current policies. Care management for people with dementia is not without its difficulties, such as balancing self-determination of the user with allowing acceptable levels of risk and ensuring that the voice of the user is heard, where articulation of their needs may be limited and the voice of the carer may seem to dominate. As mentioned previously, the Mental Capacity Act 2005 is effecting change in this respect, as this legislation assumes that vulnerable persons have the capacity to make decisions for themselves, unless it can be proved otherwise.[48]

However, this could be seen to be in conflict with the developing agenda of Safeguarding Adults policy and practice, which aims to protect 'vulnerable adults' from abuse.[49]

As previously claimed, it is argued that communication is at the heart of all approaches to dementia care, and that the need to maintain contact with others is crucial to well-being.[50] Several important issues arise from studies undertaken: firstly, the need for continuity of care, which may be difficult to achieve in some organisational contexts. Secondly, a very problematic issue is often the lack of time – one of the severe resource constraints – due to high workloads and low staff to user ratios, versus the increased amount of time needed to communicate effectively with people with dementia. Thirdly, in order to develop new person-centred approaches, staff need to acquire specialist knowledge and skills. Despite these constraints, there are promising areas of development in relation to communicating through creativity and communication with people with advanced dementia, and there is also the emergence of people with dementia relating their own experiences.[50]

Most developments in dementia care have focused on white ethnocentric approaches, and there has been limited research into the needs of ethnic minority communities in this respect. An early study by Boneham and colleagues of Black British, Afro Caribbean and Chinese older people diagnosed as suffering from dementia or depression suggested a low level of service despite considerable unmet need, due to communication difficulties, lack of knowledge of services or their culturally inappropriateness.[51] A later study by Adamson of African/Caribbean and South Asian families pointed to a lack of awareness of the condition of dementia and the need for appropriate information.[52] Both studies indicated that all the themes addressed in this chapter are exacerbated by cultural factors. An area of debate within this field is the extent to which ethnicity explains the differences of experiences of dementia among people from diverse ethnic groups. It is suggested that this might be but one of the factors, along with the degree of acculturation, socioeconomic status, education and literacy levels and household and community structures, which impact on the differences in family beliefs and attitudes about illness, dementia and caring.[53] However, a further dimension could be the issue of discrimination, as it is suggested that assessment will possibly be based on dominant white norms without adequate attention being paid to cultural differences.[54] It should, however, be pointed out that there are some good examples, such as an award-winning initiative in Bradford, involving the council, NHS Bradford and Airedale, Age Concern and the Alzheimer's Society, where a small team undertake a wide range of activities to reach out and engage with people with dementia and their carers, to deliver services and education.[55]

Although the emphasis of community care on maintaining older people in their own homes wherever possible applies equally to people suffering with dementia, it must be acknowledged that for some people this may not be possible, and a range of alternatives to home care must be considered. Although there has been no coherent joint approach between housing policy and the broader context of health and social care policies, the importance of housing is paramount in providing quality in care settings. A decade ago, a report of the Royal Commission provided a useful starting point for an analysis of possible models of supporting people in their own homes or in other settings, exploring aspects such as Intensive Home Support, Co-resident care, Very Sheltered Housing and Assistive technology. The Report also noted: 'Dementia, more than physical incapacity, can present both family members and services with particular difficulties and extreme demands.'[56]

The recommendations presented in the above report have undoubtedly led to the development of new models of housing to support people with dementia, such as dementia clusters or units within main housing schemes or a range of design features to support orientation and independence.[57] However, evidence as to the extent which these meet the needs of people with dementia is limited, and would suggest that whilst the quality of life can be enhanced for those people with mild to moderate dementia, given a range of supportive factors such as staff training, models of care and assistive technologies, they are less likely to be able to support residents as their dementia becomes more advanced.[57]

Whilst many people with dementia continue to live in their own homes or supported housing, for a significant proportion of people a move to care or nursing homes becomes inevitable. This transition can be distressing for both family carers and the person with dementia, who may not be able to recognise or accept the need for more help than the carer can provide.[58] Although the principles of person-centred care have been developing over the last 10–15 years, research suggests that this has been less evident in care homes, with the major focus being on symptom reduction and the outcomes of a range of practices.[57] Some of the main dilemmas appear to be the lack of specialist dementia training for staff, the variation in levels of healthcare and the need for more research, particularly in relation to the effects of different cultural perspectives on the quality of dementia care.

A concluding comment must be that the challenges and new directions for social care professionals working in the field of dementia care, in the current contexts of multidisciplinary policy and practice and organisational and financial constraints, must incorporate flexibility of approach and a wide range of perspectives in order to achieve good practice. The 2009 National Dementia Strategy, which is now being implemented, should be very supportive of an integrated future approach to dementia. Better information, earlier diagnosis and more memory clinics, if implemented, will give valuable support to users and carers.

Key points

➤ There are many ways of viewing ageing – sociological, physical, psychological, biological – which have influenced views of dementia.

➤ There has been a dramatic development in new ways of thinking about dementia over the last 20 years. These new ways focus on positive person-centred care, rather than a medical model.

➤ The many recent developments in community care have had limited impact on the needs of people with dementia.

➤ Services for people with dementia remain patchy, some very good, some poor.

➤ We still place a great degree of reliance on informal carers.

➤ The challenge is to use the new knowledge and the new ways of working in practice, with emphasis on interdisciplinary working and placing the user at the centre of care. This means considerable work to break down professional barriers.

➤ The 2009 National Dementia Strategy should have a positive impact on both policy and practice, although it will take time and additional resources to implement it fully.

REFERENCES

1 Alzheimer's Disease International. *World Alzheimer Report*. London: Alzheimer's Disease International; 2009.

2 Access Economics Pty Limited for Asia Pacific members of ADI. *Dementia in the Asia Pacific Region: the epidemic is here*. London: Alzheimer's Disease International; 2006.

3 Alzheimer's Society. *Dementia UK: a report into the prevalence and cost of dementia prepared by the Personal Social Services Research Unit (PSSRU) at the London School of Economics and the Institute of Psychiatry at King's College, London*. 2007 London: Alzheimer's Society; 2001. Available at: www.alzheimers.org.uk/site/scripts/download_info.php?fileID=2 (accessed August 2011).

4 Alzheimer's Society. *Dementia Awareness Week*. London: Alzheimer's Society; 2009.

5 Stephan B, Brayne C. Prevalence and projections of dementia. In: Downs M, Bowers B (eds). *Excellence in Dementia Care: research into practice*. Maidenhead: Open University Press and McGraw Hill Education; 2008.

6 Thompson N. *Age and Dignity: working with older people*. Aldershot: Arena/Ashgate Publishing Ltd; 1995.

7 Wilson K, Ruch G, Lymbery M, *et al. Social Work: an introduction to contemporary practice*. Harlow: Pearson Longman; 2008.

8 Bond J, Coleman P, Peace S. *Ageing in Society: an introduction to social gerontology*. 3rd ed. London: Sage Publications; 2007.

9 Department of Health. *The National Service Framework for Older People*. London: HMSO; 2001.

10 Department for Work and Pensions. *Link Age*, London: DWP; 2004.

11 Central Government. *Opportunity Age*. London: HMSO; 2005.

12 Department for Work and Pensions. *Building a Society for all Ages*. London: DWP; 2009.

13 Kitwood T. *Dementia Reconsidered: the person comes first*. Buckingham: Open University Press; 1997.

14 Cantley C. Understanding the policy context. In: Cantley C (ed). *A Handbook of Dementia Care*. Buckingham: Open University Press; 2001.

15 Brooker, D. *Person-centred Dementia Care: making services better*. London: Jessica Kingsley Publishers; 2007.

16 Baldwin C, Capstick A (eds). *Tom Kitwood on Dementia: a reader and critical commentary*. Maidenhead: Open University Press; 2007.

17 Innes A. *Dementia Studies*. London: Sage; 2009.

18 Moniz-Cook E, Manthorpe J (eds). *EARLY Psychosocial Interventions in Dementia: evidence-based practice*. London: Jessica Kingsley Publishers; 2009.

19 James O. *Contented Dementia*. London: Vermilion; 2008.

20 Wark P. Dementia: a new way to treat it. *The Times*, 3 August 2009.

21 Allan K, Killick J. Communication and relationships: an inclusive social world. In: Downs M, Bowers B (eds). *Excellence in Dementia Care: research into practice*. Maidenhead: Open University Press/McGraw Hill Education; 2008. pp. 212–29.

22 Morris G, Morris J. *The Dementia Care Workbook*. Maidenhead: Open University Press/McGraw Hill Education; 2010.

23 Downs M, Bowers B. *Excellence in Dementia Care: research into practice*. Maidenhead: Open University Press/McGraw Hill Education; 2008.

24 Mountain, G. Assessment and dementia. In: Downs M, Bowers B (eds). *Excellence in Dementia Care: research into practice*. Maidenhead: Open University Press/McGraw Hill Education; 2008. pp. 135–50.

25 O'Connor D, Purves B (eds). *Decision-Making, Personhood and Dementia: exploring the interface*. London: Jessica Kingsley Publishers; 2009.

26 Tibbs MA. *Social Work and Dementia: Good Practice and Care Management*. London: Jessica Kingsley Publishers; 2001. pp. 17–37.

27 Sharkey P. *The Essentials of Community Care: a guide for practitioners*. Basingstoke: Macmillan; 2007.

28 Department of Health. *Fair Access to Care Services*. London: DoH; 2002.

29 Commission for Social Care Inspection. *Cutting the Cake Fairly: CSCI review of eligibility criteria for social care*. London: CSCI; 2008.

30 Department of Health. *Putting People First*. London: DoH; 2007.

31 Department of Health. *Shaping the Future of Care Together*. London: DoH; 2009.

32 Audit Commission. *Forget Me Not: mental health services for older people*. London: Audit Commission; 2000.

33 Audit Commission Update *Forget Me Not 2002*. London: Audit Commission; 2002.

34 National Institute for Health and Clinical Excellence. *Dementia: supporting people with dementia and their carers in health and social care. NICE guideline 42*. London: NICE. www.nice.org.uk/guidance/GCO42 (2006, modified 2011).

35 Alzheimer's Society. *Dementia UK*. London: Alzheimer's Society; 2007.

36 National Audit Office. *Improving Services and Support for People with Dementia*. London: NAO; 2007.

37 Department of Health. *End of Life Strategy*. London: DoH; 2008.

38 Department of Health. *Living Well with Dementia: a National Dementia Strategy*. London: DoH; 2009.

39 Seddon D, Robinson C. Carers of older people with dementia: assessment and the Carers Act. *Health and Social Care in the Community*. 2001; 9(3): 151–8.

40 Department of Health. *Caring about Carers: a National Strategy for Carers*. London: HMSO; 1999.

41 Nolan M, Keady J. Working with carers. In: Cantley C (ed). *A Handbook of Dementia Care*. Buckingham: Open University Press; 2001.

42 Department of Health. *Carers Grant 2008–2011 Best Practice Guidance*. London: DoH; 2008.

43 Netten A. The costs of informal care. In: Clark C, Lapsley I (eds). *Planning and Costing Community Care*. London: Jessica Kingsley Publishers; 1996.

44 Orme J. *Gender and Community Care: social work and social care perspectives*. Basingstoke: Palgrave; 2001. pp. 99, 168.

45 Heron C. *Working with Carers*. London: Jessica Kingsley Publishers; 1998.

46 Whitman L (ed). *Telling Tales about Dementia*. London: Jessica Kingsley Publishers; 2010.

47 Millen J, Wallman-Durrant L. Multi-disciplinary partnership in a community mental health team. In: White V, Harris J (eds). *Developing Good Practice in Community Care: partnership and participation*. London: Jessica Kingsley Publishers; 2001.

48 Mountain G. Assessment and dementia. In: Downs M, Bowers B (eds). *Excellence in Dementia Care: research into practice*. Maidenhead: Open University Press/McGraw Hill Education; 2008.

49 Mantell A, Scragg T. *Safeguarding Adults in Social Work*. Exeter: Learning Matters; 2008.

50 Killick J, Allan K. Communication and relationships. In: Downs M, Bowers B (eds). *Excellence in Dementia Care: research into practice*. Maidenhead: Open University Press/McGraw Hill Education; 2008.

51 Boneham MA, Williams KE, Copeland JRM, *et al.* Elderly people from ethnic minorities in Liverpool: mental illness, unmet need and barriers to service use. *Health and Social Care in the Community*. 1997; 5(3): 173–80.

52 Adamson J. Awareness and understanding of dementia in African/Caribbean and South Asian families. *Health and Social Care in the Community*. 2001; 9(6): 391–6.

53 Boise L. Ethnicity and the experience of dementia. In: Downs M, Bowers B (eds). *Excellence in Dementia Care: research into practice*. Maidenhead: Open University Press/McGraw Hill Education; 2008.

54 Thompson N. *Anti-discriminatory Practice*. 4th ed. Basingstoke: Palgrave Macmillan; 2006.

55 Metropolitan District of Bradford Council. *Meri Yaadain*. Bradford: Metropolitan District of Bradford Council; 2009.

56 Royal Commission on Long Term Care for Elderly People. *With Respect to Old Age: long term care – rights and responsibilities*. vol. 2. London: HMSO; 1999. p. 178.

57 Evans S, Vallelly S, Croucher K. The role of specialist housing in supporting older people with dementia. In: Downs M, Bowers B (eds). *Excellence in Dementia Care: research into practice*. Maidenhead: Open University Press/McGraw Hill Education; 2008.

58 Fossey J. Care homes. In: Downs M, Bowers B (eds). *Excellence in Dementia Care: research into practice*. Maidenhead: Open University Press/McGraw Hill Education; 2008.

CHAPTER 11

Towards practical service delivery for younger people with dementia

Tony Dearden
(revised for this edition by the editors)

INTRODUCTION

In recent years there has been a growing recognition that younger people with dementia and their carers can have very different needs to older people and that existing health and social care provision is very poorly adjusted to accommodate these differences. The historical division of health and social services, based upon the age of 65 years, has often resulted in patients, and carers, being marooned between general psychiatry, old age psychiatry and neurology.

Addressing the needs of early onset dementia sufferers, that is, those people with dementia who are under 65 years of age, and their families, presents a serious organisational challenge to all agencies. In addition, the early onset dementias are a very heterogeneous group of disorders with widely varying presentations, quite different cognitive and physical impairments as well as a wide range of psychiatric and behavioural features, which will challenge any clinical team. The aims of this chapter are to summarise the key issues, both clinical and organisational, as space does not allow for detailed discussion. However, it is the intention to indicate where improvements to clinical care should and can be made, based on published evidence and practical experience.

DIFFERENCES?

The management of younger patients can present different problems because of their different social, economic and family circumstances. The ways in which the needs of younger people may differ from those over 65 include the following.

➤ Younger people are more likely to be in work at the time of diagnosis.

➤ Carers of younger people with dementia are likely to face different life conditions to carers of older people.

➤ Younger people are likely to be more active than older people, their physical strength may be greater and behaviour may be more problematic.

➤ Younger people are more likely to have dependent children and heavy financial commitments.

➤ They experience different emotional reactions. For both the person with dementia and their family, the diagnosis has a dramatic effect on future life plans and expectations.[1]

Genetic aspects and the issue of inheritance are of greater concern and more common. There is a higher prevalence of the 'rarer dementias' and clinicians need the awareness, knowledge and experience to work with the different needs presented by the whole range of dementias.

However, it is important to recognise that the 'age 65 cut-off' is biological nonsense and that people experience a continuum of physical, psychological and social changes. There are also a great many similarities between dementia in younger and older people, the key principles of good quality care are the same, and the knowledge and skills used in one area of practice can be transferred to another.

THE EXPERIENCE OF PEOPLE WITH EARLY ONSET DEMENTIA AND THEIR FAMILIES

There have been a number of local studies in different parts of the UK assessing the needs of younger people with dementia. A review of the literature reveals the main areas of concern to most, if not all, sufferers, carers and service providers to be as follows.

Difficulties in assessing the numbers and levels of demand

Alternative methods of determining prevalence and incidence have produced widely varying figures. This has resulted in uncertainty, with service providers anxious that resources will be insufficient for the demand and commissioners reluctant to invest in the development of a service that might subsequently be underused. Fortunately there is now an adequate evidence base and a lot of practical experience from around the country that enables clinicians and managers to predict the numbers and quantify the likely service needs of a local population (see below).

Poor service articulation and co-ordination

The relatively low prevalence and incidence of early onset dementia means that there are often no clearly articulated pathways to appropriate diagnosis, assessment and aftercare existing for this client group. Referrals for diagnosis are made to a diverse range of health professionals, including neurologists, psychiatrists, psychologists and physicians. As a result, people frequently end up receiving either no care at all in the initial stages of dementia or widely differing packages of care. People with dementia and their carers can be left unsupported for some time after diagnosis, and only after a crisis point has been reached do support services become involved.

Problems with information and advice

Patients and carers frequently report that insufficient information is given at, and after, diagnosis regarding the nature of the illness and the availability of support services. Great sensitivity is needed to determine how much information people are ready to receive and when it is appropriate to give such information and advice. Carers and sufferers need information about the illness and its effects, financial and legal advice, information on available health, social and voluntary sector provision, and advice on coping with psychiatric and behavioural problems.

Inappropriate support services

Younger people with dementia are frequently reluctant to receive elderly services when they are provided because they feel that they do not belong in a setting where other users are usually very much older and less active than they are. Similarly, under-65 adult mental health services are usually intended for people with very different needs and are rarely able to provide the degree of supervision required by people with dementia, resulting in the danger of younger people being 'orphaned in a no man's land' between services.

The burden of coping

Early onset dementia is characterised by a high psychiatric and behavioural morbidity compared with late onset dementia.[2,3] These non-cognitive symptoms are particularly stressful to carers, and research has shown them to be even more strongly associated with care-giver burden than other very powerful influences such as the degree of impairment and the duration of dementia.[4,5] These very high levels of carer burden are thought in turn to lead to greater levels of service use.

HOW MANY?

As someone involved for some time in developing services for younger people with dementia, I have heard many clinicians express concerns that they would become overburdened by the number of patients (high) whilst at the same time listening to managers express concerns that they could not justify investment for the number of people involved (low). Therefore, the availability of reasonably accurate estimates of the frequency of early onset dementia, i.e. incidence and prevalence data, should help remove some of the uncertainty and anxiety for health service planners, managers and clinicians and encourage the development of needs-led and cost-effective services.

The different methodologies employed by researchers and clinicians in the various epidemiological and local needs assessment studies have produced in the literature a wide range in the rates of prevalence and incidence in any given population. However, the larger studies with good case definition and sampling methods do give very similar findings. What follows is not intended to be a scientific exposition of the complex epidemiological issues, but the headline information and evidence that should be useful to those developing services.

Research by Newens et al.,[6] investigating Alzheimer's disease only, reported a prevalence of 34.6 per 100 000 people between the ages of 45 and 64 years. This finding has been replicated by Harvey,[2] who reported a rate of 35 per 100 000 for the same age range. The same study also examined the rates of other causes of early onset dementia in two London boroughs and a summary of this population by type of dementia is shown in Figure 11.1.

It can be seen that only one in three cases of early onset dementia is due to Alzheimer's disease, a significantly lower proportion than in later life. Many

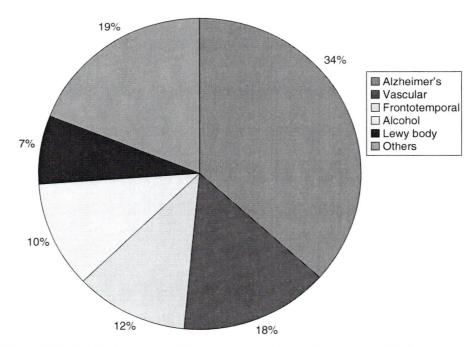

Figure 11.1 Relative prevalence of different types of dementia in younger people

clinicians working in this field have found even lower rates than quoted for Lewy body dementia, a very common condition amongst 70 and 80-year-olds with dementia. In contrast, frontotemporal lobar dementia accounts for one in seven cases of early onset dementia, although it appears to be underdiagnosed in clinical practice. It has three subcategories: frontotemporal dementia, semantic dementia and progressive non-fluent aphasia. Alcoholic dementia is a condition of the relatively young and it can be seen that a much higher proportion of cases compared with older adults are due to other causes. The most common and important other causes include Huntingdon's disease, dementia in multiple sclerosis, corticobasal degeneration, connective tissue diseases, metabolic disorders, neurosyphilis, normal pressure hydrocephalus and prion diseases.

Given that the numbers of people with the non-Alzheimer's dementias are inevitably small, the frequency rates reported are less reliable and less consistent. However, the epidemiological study by Harvey[2] found the prevalence rate for all causes of dementia in 45–64 year-olds to be 98 per 100 000. This is compatible with other epidemiological work – therefore I recommend to planners as a 'good rule of thumb' to determine the number of cases in their local population, using the figure of 1 per 1000 in 45–64 year-olds.

Dementia is very rare before the age of 45 years with around 10% of early onset cases occurring before this age, mostly caused by rare and unusual diseases. Plotting the number of cases of dementia against age produces an exponential curve (*see* Figure 11.2), exemplified by the prevalence and incidence of

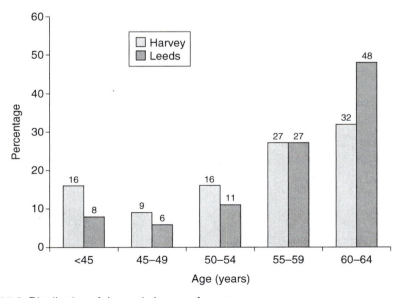

Figure 11.2 Distribution of dementia by age of onset

Alzheimer's disease, which approximately doubles every five years from the age of 40 years onwards.

Studies of risk factors in early onset dementia have investigated genetic and environmental factors. There is now a huge body of literature on the genetics and molecular pathology of Alzheimer's disease in particular. The abnormal genes identified in the dementias are summarised in Table 11.1.

Some authors have speculated that all cases of early onset Alzheimer's disease might be inherited as an autosomal dominant trait, notwithstanding that many cases have no family history. A number of studies then attempted to determine the proportion of familial cases and to assess the relative risk of dementia in the relatives of probands. The most extensive survey, to date, of a population-based series of 101 familial and sporadic cases of early onset AD, applying modern molecular genetic techniques to screen for mutations, showed an overall prevalence for mutations of only 7%: 6% presenilin-1 and 1% presenilin-2 with no cases of APP mutations.[7] When only those with a clear family history were included in the analyses, the prevalence of mutations rose to 18%. These data suggest that the identified gene mutations for Alzheimer's disease are rare and account for less than one-fifth of cases with a family history.

Table 11.1 Abnormal genes identified in the dementias

	Gene	*Chromosome*
Alzheimer's disease	Amyloid precursor protein (mutations)	21
	Presenilin-1 (mutations)	14
	Presenilin-2 (mutations)	1
Creutzfeldt–Jakob disease	Prion protein: PRNP (mutations)	20
Frontotemporal dementia	Tau (mutations)	17
Huntingdon's disease	Huntingdon (CAG trinucleotide expansion)	4

DIAGNOSIS AND ASSESSMENT

In practice, the experienced clinician can make a diagnosis in two ways. Both involve taking a history and informant history, with the aim of establishing the mode of onset, evolution and pattern and impact of any deficits, together with mental state examination, cognitive assessment, neuropsychological testing, physical examination, investigations and neuroimaging. The first method is 'pattern recognition'. That is, based on experience and knowledge of different disorders, do these symptoms and signs match any patient/syndrome I have previously seen? Do the different pieces of the jigsaw, history to neuroimaging, fit together into a meaningful whole? The second method is 'systematic analysis'. This is based on two fundamental facts: that cerebral diseases do not affect the brain uniformly, but preferentially affect certain brain regions and spare others, and that mental/psychological processes themselves are region-ally organised and depend upon the functioning of specific brain regions. It follows, therefore, that the causative disease or pathology can be deduced after the precise neuropsychological deficits have been determined.

Four main groups of patients are seen: the worried-well, the psychiatri-cally ill (particularly depression), those with a degenerative dementia and a miscellaneous group (with focal brain pathologies, delirium, etc.). The first aim of identifying the worried-well is often made more complicated because the worry is generated by a positive family history. For a significant number, follow-up over time will be the only way of making absolutely sure that subtle complaints do not herald the onset of an organic syndrome.

The proportion of cases with a potentially reversible disorder will vary according to referral patterns. Numerous systemic disorders can potentially give rise to cognitive impairment, and so it is important to take a detailed past history to see if any candidates turn up. Of particular importance are mark-ers of vasculitis such as rash, arthritis or renal disease and metabolic disorder, e.g. autoimmune thyroid disease. The traditional infection related to cognitive impairment, syphilis, is now rare in the western world but still occurs occasion-ally. HIV and its complications, e.g. progressive multifocal leukoencephalopa-thy, is now the leading infectious cause of chronic cognitive impairment.

The most common treatable differential diagnosis of degenerative dementia is psychiatric illness, particularly depression. Symptoms of mood disturbance (anhedonia, pessimistic ruminations, suicidal ideas) and biological features of depression (anorexia, early morning waking, reduced libido) should be sought in all cases. It is important to note, however, that a significant number of those with organic brain disorders will exhibit concurrent psychiatric symptoms, par-ticularly features of depression. Follow-up may be the only way of separating depression with cognitive symptoms from dementia with prominent affective symptoms.

For those who show evidence of organic impairment of cognition, the aim is to reach a specific diagnosis. A useful subclassification is into those with a relatively pure cognitive syndrome and those with associated neurological signs. The clinical patterns for the major degenerative dementias are sum-marised in Table 11.2.[8]

Difficulties in obtaining a diagnosis of dementia appear to be greater before the age of 65 years. Yet, an early diagnosis is important since it enables patient, family and carers to have a greater understanding of the illness and progno-sis, and a better opportunity to attend to work and family responsibilities and to plan the management of the illness and for the future. Delayed diagnosis causes distress for patients and the families of people with dementia. An Aus-tralian study reported that the diagnostic process was considered problematic by 71% of carers, with 21% reporting misdiagnosis, the mean time to diagnosis

Table 11.2 Clinical patterns for the major degenerative dementias

	Memory	Language	Visuospatial	Attention	Frontal behavioural symptoms	Neurological signs
Alzheimer's disease	+++	++	++	++	+/–	–
Alzheimer's: biparietal variant	+/++	+	++++	++	+/–	–
Dementia with Lewy bodies	++	+	+++	+++	+/–	++
Frontotemporal dementia – (unless associated with MND)						
Semantic dementia	+	++++	+/–	+	++	
Frontal variant	+	+	+/–	++	+++	
Progressive aphasia	+/–	+++	+/–	+	+	
Corticobasal degeneration	+	+	+++	++	++	+++
Progressive supranuclear palsy	+	+	+	+++	++	+++
Huntingdon's disease	+	+	+	+++	++	+++

MND = motor neurone disease

was 3.4 years, and that the diagnosis was only made after patients had seen an average of 2.8 health service professionals.[9] Diagnosis is more easily missed when not suspected because of patient age, when symptoms are denied by patient, family and colleagues, when symptoms are misdiagnosed as due to functional disorders,[10] or when behavioural or personality changes are the first symptoms, as they are in certain dementia syndromes.

Every patient then requires a comprehensive assessment of needs and risks in order to produce an individual care plan tailored to specific needs to enhance quality of life. This should include determining functional ability and impact upon daily living as well as the presence of particular problems, such as driving safety and risk, which applies to a much greater proportion of patients than in a service for older people. The needs assessment must also identify action required for financial support and benefits, activities, personal care, hygiene, feeding and housing. Clinical staff must also assess eligibility for treatment with cholinesterase inhibitors, or the use of other psychiatric medications, e.g. antidepressants, and the appropriateness of behavioural and psychotherapeutic management. Families and carers also need to be interviewed with a particular reference to assessment of their mental and physical health and coping styles.

INFORMATION, CARE AND SUPPORT

It can be difficult for doctors to know how much information to give to the person with dementia and their family. Professionals are often fearful of giving the diagnosis of dementia: 'it will be too upsetting' or 'there is no treatment'. The danger is that very limited information or false reassurance can make caring and planning even more stressful.

There is no doubt that the person with dementia has 'the right to know'. In practice, most people with early onset dementia, in the early stages of the disease, know there is something wrong. The commonest fears are that they are going mad, or have a brain tumour. If giving the diagnosis is handled sensitively and positively, with the assurance of long-term support and help, then it is rarely as devastating as the person giving it imagines it will be, and people are relieved to know the diagnosis. If the diagnosis is made early enough and shared, the person with dementia can play a very active part in the planning of their future care.

Sometimes people do not wish to know the name of their illness, and sometimes they deny it when it is given. In these situations, it is accepted that someone has a right not to have the name forced on them. It is important to explain the cause of the memory impairment and other cognitive, emotional and personality changes occurring as a consequence of brain changes. Often the knowledge that repetitive questioning or conversation, emotional changes, lack of care and concern, loss of skills, poor personal hygiene and poor recent memory are due to a disease process, and not wilful 'awkwardness', is in many ways a relief.

The person giving the diagnosis should emphasise the positive aspects of what can be done to help the person with dementia and others, as well as giving an account of the specific illness and the course it is likely to take. The course and rate of progression of dementia varies dramatically between different diseases. Older patients with Alzheimer's disease may live for up to 20 years; in younger patients the dementia will generally progress at a faster rate, while patients with frontotemporal dementia and motor neurone disease will have a life expectancy of only a few months. Several epidemiological studies report survival data for their cohorts.[6,11] These data suggest that approaching 50% of patients with early onset AD will have died within five years, with a lower survival rate for vascular dementia. There is some evidence to show that the presence of tremor, rigidity or myoclonus is associated with significantly reduced survival at five years after diagnosis.

All of this information is far too much to share in one or even two sessions and needs to be dealt with gradually, in the context of a trusting, supportive relationship, over a period of weeks or months. It is important to give patients the opportunity to discuss their feelings and queries at a later date. They should know that support and help will be ongoing, and that help will be on hand to address both psychological and practical difficulties in the time ahead. The knowledge that there is someone on hand to help with everyday problems, who understands both the person with early onset dementia and carer experience, is in itself usually an enormous help.

Taking a problem-oriented approach is the most effective means of helping the person with early onset dementia and their carer. Helping the person with dementia and their carer to break the illness down into problems that can have a solution, rather than a progressive, degenerative disease, is a much more positive and helpful approach, which, if started early enough in the illness, can significantly relieve stress. It is then possible to see often very distressing symptoms as part of an illness process, which can in turn be addressed in a structured manner. It is also possible to tackle problems not due to dementia, many of which can be remedied.

The other therapeutic aspect of the counselling relationship is in helping the person with dementia and their family come to terms with the changes in their lives, with the losses that have occurred and those still to come. The changes forced upon carers are often considerable, for example, changes in financial circumstances with many carers still having large financial commitments such as mortgages, and many carers having to reduce working hours or stop work altogether. In one investigation 90% had financial problems.[9] The same study reported a severe impact on children, with 92% significantly affected by the dementia. Emotional problems, problems at school and conflict with the person with dementia were described. Two major predictors of both increased psychological distress and burden frequently reported in studies are poor marital quality pre-diagnosis and a female carer.

DEVELOPING SERVICES

Strategic and financial planning should be informed by research and the experiences of people with dementia and their carers, together with clinical experience combined with the evaluation of services.

The Leeds Service has been developing incrementally since 1995 and currently comprises the following.

➤ The early onset dementia (EOD) team – with sessional time from a consultant psychiatrist, a consultant clinical psychologist, a full-time community mental health nurse, two half-time social workers, one full-time occupational therapist and a full-time secretary. The team works mostly in the community but also runs an outpatient clinic.

➤ Armley Grange Day Centre – run by the Alzheimer's Society, open five days per week, providing places per day specifically for younger people with dementia. Day care has been rated the most valuable service consistently by carers in many surveys in the UK, e.g. Williams *et al.*[12]

➤ A group for younger people with dementia and groups for carers.

➤ A new outreach service staffed by the Alzheimer's Society, taking referrals from the EOD team to provide additional domiciliary care and help maintain people in their home setting. This focuses on the individual's strengths and provides opportunities for interesting and stimulating activities in the home or the wider community.

➤ Dedicated beds on a dementia acute ward and agreed access to respite and continuing care beds in a NHS community unit for older people with dementia.

Where specialist provision does not exist then generic services such as home care and Crossroads (a charity providing home-based respite care) are used, as are health services, social services and independent sector services designed for other client groups, e.g. residential and nursing homes for older people with dementia.

Development requires multi-agency working with professionals collaborating across agencies, e.g. clinicians with commissioners and the voluntary sector. Based upon personal experience, I suggest the following 10 key messages.[13]

1 Examine current provision.

2 Adapt and develop around existing services.

3 Learn from other people.

4 Plan and be prepared for a long and frustrating process.

5 Set clear aims and objectives.

6 Create political alliances and involve people capable of effecting organisational change.

7 Identify named professionals and 'product champions'.

8 Involve carers – their voice can be very powerful.

9 Involve people with dementia – as above.

10 Action – make a start somewhere! Changing the whole system has to be done in steps.

I have found that even experienced CPNs and specialist registrars find working with younger people extremely challenging, due to the emotional impact of speaking to people of a similar age to themselves about having a diagnosis, together with the complexity of need and severity of behavioural problems. The need for building in supervision and support to staff as well as providing training cannot be overstated. Suggested topics for training include:

➤ understanding the symptoms and signs of the rarer dementias

➤ breaking of bad news

➤ responding to difficult questions.

A COMPREHENSIVE SERVICE MODEL

Any service model should have as its ethos 'joint working' across the whole system of care. A close working relationship between the different service providers is an essential foundation, as is multidisciplinary teamwork, if complex needs are to be met in a coherent and co-ordinated manner. The following issues are critical:

➤ early and accurate diagnosis

➤ access for all younger people with dementia to a full range of quality services

➤ services which reflect the specific needs and circumstances of younger people

➤ services that are financially justifiable and sustainable.

A study by the Alzheimer's Society found 11 pathways to care[14] and another demonstrated 38 different referral pathways to care.[12] A clear link between neurology services and mental health services goes some way to avoiding the need to negotiate a maze of services.

The Royal College of Psychiatrists proposes that each district should have one named consultant responsible for the service, suggesting old age psychiatrists are best placed to fulfil this role, whilst the task force initiated by the European Federation of Neurological Societies recommends that neurologists should have a clear role in the management of dementia. A 2002 survey to assess then current stated practice in the UK in the diagnosis and management of younger people with dementia confirmed some previously reported differences between old age psychiatrists and neurologists.[15]

It is important to know that neurologists and old age psychiatrists investigate and manage patients differently, especially given that neurologists manage patients without liaison with old age psychiatrists and vice versa. Significantly more old age psychiatrists obtained an independent history from a carer, assessed symptoms of depression and changes in driving performance, arranged community follow-up and prescribed and monitored acetylcholinesterase inhibitor therapy. Significantly more neurologists performed physical examinations and arranged more basic investigations, e.g. plasma viscosity, syphilis serology, EEG, as well as more specialist investigations such as lumbar puncture for examination of CSF. Neuroimaging has an increasingly sophisticated part to play in diagnosis (*see* Chapter 4 on page 57 *et seq.*).

Young patients may be underinvestigated if managed by an old age psychiatrist and may not receive adequate follow-up services if managed solely by a neurologist. The assessment and management of patients with early onset dementia would be greatly improved if the complementary skills of both neurologists and old age psychiatrists were employed in the care of each patient. A joint assessment clinic is probably the best way of facilitating this, but where it does not exist patients should be speedily referred from the diagnostic service to the community mental health team, so as to provide emotional support early. Psychiatrists ought to refer all patients with atypical presentations and those under 50 years old to a neurologist.

The preferred model of care is a named care co-ordinator (from the EOD team) supervising an integrated package of health and social care tailored to individual needs, providing continuity and reviewing changing needs, in other words a Care Programme Approach (CPA) model or equivalent. A community mental health team is the focal point, networked to other services such as day care, respite services and acute hospital services.

There is now a lot of practical experience and an adequate evidence base that demonstrates the need for specialist service provision. This can then streamline the diagnostic process, clarify clinical responsibility, build up expertise, provide continuity and co-ordinate the delivery of care with other agencies.

THE FUTURE

Following the inclusion of younger people with dementia in the National Service Framework for Older People[16] and various reports, including one from the National Audit Office,[17] the National Dementia Strategy for England[18] (and its equivalents for Scotland, Wales and Northern Ireland) was published in 2009. This is discussed in more detail in Chapter 1. The objectives of this Strategy apply to people of all ages with dementia. Objective 2 of the Strategy (good quality early diagnosis and intervention), objective 3 (good quality information) and objective 4 (access to a dementia advisor) are particularly relevant. The dementia advisor will need to be trained to take into account the special needs of people with early onset dementia. The implementation of the Strategy should give scope for the inclusion of younger people within general dementia services. Nevertheless, unless a specialist service is retained it will remain essential to train some team members specifically to address the needs of younger people.

Key points

➤ The practical management of younger people with dementia requires attention to both the clinical challenge, e.g. of diagnosis and psychiatric management, and the organisational challenge of how to design and co-ordinate a range of services.

➤ It is this author's hope and prediction that more new services will be set up and that the existing knowledge base will fully inform clinical practice and management.

REFERENCES

1 Alzheimer's Disease Society. *Younger People with Dementia: a review and Strategy.* London: ADS; 1996. See also www.alzheimers.org.uk/factsheet/440 (accessed May 2011).

2 Harvey R. *Young Onset Dementia: epidemiology, clinical symptoms, family burden, support and outcome.* London: Imperial College School of Medicine; 1998.

3 Ferran J, Wilson K, Doran M, *et al.* The early-onset dementias: a study of clinical characteristics and service use. *International Journal of Geriatric Psychiatry.* 1996; **11**: 863–9.

4 Donaldson C, Tarrier N, Burns A. The impact of the symptoms of dementia on caregivers. *British Journal of Psychiatry.* 1997; **170**: 62–8.

5 Teri L. Behaviour and care-giver burden: behavioural problems in patients with Alzheimer disease and its association with care-giver distress. *Alzheimer Disease and Associated Disorders.* 1997; **11**: S35–S38.

6 Newens A, Forster D, Kay D, *et al.* Clinically diagnosed presenile dementia of the Alzheimer type in the Northern region: ascertainment, prevalence, incidence and survival. *Psychological Medicine.* 1993; **23**: 631–44.

7 Cruts M, Vanduijn CM, Backhovens H, *et al.* Estimation of the genetic contribution of presenilin-1 and -2 mutations in a population-based study of pre-senile Alzheimer's disease. *Human Molecular Genetics.* 1998; **7**: 43–51.

8 Hodges JR (ed). *Early Onset Dementia: a multidisciplinary approach.* Oxford: Oxford University Press; 2001.

9 Luscombe G, Brodaty H, Freeth S. Younger people with dementia: diagnostic issues, effects on carers and use of services. *International Journal of Geriatric Psychiatry*. 1998; **13**: 323–30.

10 Nott P, Fleminger J. Presenile dementia: the difficulties of early diagnosis. *Acta Psychiatrica Scandinavica*. 1975; **51**:210–17.

11 Whalley L, Thomas B, McGonigal G, *et al*. Epidemiology of pre-senile Alzheimer's disease in Scotland (1974–1988). *British Journal of Psychiatry*. 1995; **167**: 728–31.

12 Williams T, Dearden AM, Cameron IC. From pillar to post: a study of younger people with dementia. *Psychiatric Bulletin*. 2001; **25**: 384–7.

13 Alzheimer's Disease Society. *Younger People with Dementia: a guide to service development and provision*. London: ADS; 2001.

14 Fuhrmann R. *Early Onset Dementia in the Brighton, Hove and Lewes Area: prevalence and service needs*. Brighton: Alzheimer's Society; 1997.

15 Cordery R, Harvey R, Frost C, *et al*. National survey to assess current practices in the diagnosis and management of young people with dementia. *International Journal of Geriatric Psychiatry*. 2002; **17**: 124–7.

16 Department of Health. *National Service Framework for Older People*. London: DoH; 2001.

17 National Audit Office. *Improving Services and Support for People with Dementia*. London: NAO; 2007.

18 Department of Health. *Living Well with Dementia: a National Strategy*. London: DoH; 2009.

FURTHER READING

➤ Cox S, Keady J (eds). *Younger People with Dementia: planning, practice and development*. London: Jessica Kingsley Publishers; 1999.

➤ Neary D. Classification of the dementias. *Reviews in Clinical Gerontology*. 1994; **4**: 131–40.

➤ Royal College of Psychiatrists. *Services for Younger People with Alzheimer's Disease and Other Dementias*. Council Report No. 77. London: Royal College of Psychiatrists; 2000.

➤ Williams R, Barrett K, Muth Z (eds). *Mental Health Services: heading for better care – commissioning and providing mental health services for people with Huntingdon's disease, acquired brain injury and early-onset dementia*. NHS Health Advisory Service thematic review. London: HMSO; 1997.

➤ Williams T, Cameron I, Dearden T, *et al*. *From Pillar to Post: early-onset dementia in Leeds – prevalence, experience and service need*. Leeds: Leeds Health Authority; 1999.

CHAPTER 12

Understanding behavioural change in dementia

Elizabeth Milwain

BRAIN, BEHAVIOUR AND DEMENTIA

Damage to the brain can cause predictable changes in behaviour. Damage to the under-surfaces of the frontal lobe is known to cause dramatic changes in personality,[1] whilst damage to the outer surfaces, especially on the left side, is associated with apathy.[2] Reductions in the availability of the neurotransmitter serotonin within the cerebral cortex is associated with aggression.[3] It can be tempting, therefore, to think that brain damage is the main cause of behavioural change in dementia.

Proponents of person-centred approaches argue strongly that this approach is too narrow. In his book *Dementia Reconsidered*,[4] Tom Kitwood wrote:

> If we follow the development of any person's dementing condition closely, again and again we will come to see how social and interpersonal factors come into play, either by adding to the difficulties arising from neurological impairment, or helping to lessen their effects. In light of this it is extremely difficult to hold the view suggested by the standard paradigm: that the mental and emotional symptoms are a direct result of a catastrophic series of changes in the brain that lead to the death of nerve cells – and nothing more than that.
>
> (p. 40)

The aim of this chapter is to use knowledge from neuropsychology, particularly with regard to changing memory functions, to illustrate how the neurological, the psychological and the social can interact to affect a person's behaviour. It is hoped that this will support Kitwood's argument and caution the reader against an overly narrow approach to understanding the role of brain damage in behavioural change in dementia. There is, however, a complementary danger within person-centred approaches of neglecting the neurological element and assuming it is of lesser value in explaining behavioural change relative to psychological and social influences. It is hoped that the illustration provided will also demonstrate that an understanding of the neurological element of dementia is as crucial to understanding the person with dementia as are the psychological and social elements.

THE NATURE OF MEMORY BREAKDOWN IN ALZHEIMER'S DISEASE

The discussion in this chapter is intended as an illustration and not as a framework that will apply to every person with dementia. The focus is specifically upon the neuropathology of Alzheimer's disease, the impact of that pathology on memory functions and how, in turn, this may affect behaviour. Alzheimer's disease is the most common cause of dementia and is involved either on its own or in conjunction with other causes in up to 85% of cases.[5] The illustration should, therefore, have relevance for a significant majority of people with dementia.

Memory loss is the cardinal symptom of Alzheimer's disease. Prominent symptoms of this disorder revolve around memory failures, such as forgetting the shopping, forgetting conversations, forgetting appointments, forgetting visits from family and so forth. The aim of this chapter is not to list all the many different consequences of memory loss but rather to use knowledge about the nature and organisation of the memory system to try to understand how the world might look if this system were subject to partial but progressive damage. This deeper insight into how memory loss may change the person's whole understanding of the world about them allows for a better understanding of a range of behaviours which would otherwise seem illogical and bizarre.

In most people with Alzheimer's disease the hippocampus (shown in Figure 12.1), together with some smaller structures on the inner rim of the temporal lobe, becomes the neural cradle within which the disease process takes hold and gains strength.[6,7] These structures have long been known to have a crucial role in memory formation,[8] and the early damage here explains those common early problems with forgetting the shopping, conversations, visits, appointments and so forth. From this cradle, the disease process spreads out to affect a number of different areas within the cerebral cortex. The cerebral cortex covers the surfaces of the two cerebral hemispheres (*see* Figure 12.1) and accounts for 80% of the brain's total volume.[9] It provides the brain's main source of processing power and performs a number of complex functions relating to conscious perception, understanding and the planning and control of behaviour. Accumulating damage to the cortex sees the decline of the associated intellectual functions (for a more detailed review of the effects of damage to the cerebral cortex see Perrin *et al.*[10]).

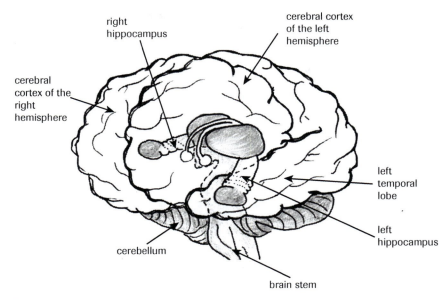

The cerebral cortex is a thin sheet of nerve cells that covers the surface of both the left and right cerebral hemispheres. The areas of the sheet that cover the temporal lobes are particularly important for memory functions. Only the left temporal lobe can be seen in this diagram, but the right temporal lobe occupies the corresponding position on the opposite side.

Figure 12.1 The approximate position of the hippocampus and cerebral cortex within the human brain

The following discussion tracks the cognitive effects of the progression from the hippocampal cradle to the first forays into the cerebral cortex, and corresponds to the early to mid stages of the disease. Together the hippocampus and cerebral cortex of the temporal lobe provide a powerful memory system for the formation and storage of what are termed declarative memories; memories that can be consciously accessed, thought about, reflected upon and shared with others through language.[11] Declarative memories are further subdivided into episodic and semantic traces.[12] In an episodic trace the content of a learning experience remains connected to the time and place of learning and is encoded as a unique and specific event (e.g. memory for the first day at school). In a semantic trace the content is not tied to a specific time and place, but encodes knowledge about some kind of thing or event which is repeatedly experienced (e.g. knowing what a cat is, knowing Paris is the capital of France, knowing how to behave in a restaurant).

Within this declarative memory system the hippocampus is the gateway to all new declarative learning. It is understood to provide the mechanism by which all the different sensory aspects of an experience can be fused into a single whole to create an instant and complex record of an experience, tagging the content to the time and place of occurrence.[13] Initially, therefore, all new memories are episodic in nature. Evidence suggests, however, that the hippocampus provides only temporary storage and that the bonds to time and place information decay over time (see Groeger[14] for a review). New learning is retained for the longer term only if it is consolidated to the 'archiving' networks, which have been located primarily to the cortex of the temporal lobe.[15]

Research into autobiographical memory shows that for normal subjects memories from both the earliest and the latest decades of life are most readily recalled, but that memories from the middle decades are harder to access. Mackinnon and Squire[16] asked subjects to think of autobiographical memories in response to 75 cues such as tree, flag or window. The people interviewed recalled an average of 15 memories from 40 years or more ago, compared with only five memories from the period of either 20–30 or 10–20 years ago. However, whilst normal subjects recalled an average of 15 memories from the most recent period of up to 10 years ago, patients with hippocampal damage remembered very few recent experiences from this time period. On the basis of these findings, and other research into the nature of memory consolidation, it is hypothesised that it takes a period of up to two years for memories to be effectively transferred from the hippocampal to the cortical memory system[17] and that, generally, older memories are consolidated more firmly than newer ones.

One of the factors involved in consolidation, as might be expected, is repetition.[18,19] However, even when repetition is taken into account, the age at which a memory was acquired seems to exert an additional force in strengthening a memory. Ellis *et al.*[20] suggest part of the consolidation process is not the mere repetition of material, but the integration of new material with existing knowledge. Indeed, it has long been known that this kind of integration is the most efficient way to learn new information.[21,22] The earliest acquired knowledge seems to form the base into which all subsequent knowledge is woven, giving it a particularly rich set of connections within the whole system. This may explain why childhood and adolescent memories are so enduring, together with the fact that special, distinctive emotions are often experienced the first time something is done, helping to differentiate that first time from all subsequent times.

Childhood memories are examples of memories in which the whole memory, complete with information about the learning context, is transferred into the archives. These memories retain their episodic characteristics through time. As noted above, such events tend to be either distinctive or emotionally arousing. It is not immediately obvious how the principle of repetition operates here, given that such events, by definition, can only be experienced once. However, when an event is recalled from its temporary storage in the hippocampus, it is remembered by being replayed through the networks of the cortex involved in the perception and understanding of the original event.[23] Replay not only gives the 'lived again' experience, but also repeats the pattern across the cortex, strengthening the record in the long-term archives. Important events are also repeated by telling other people about the experience. Part of the retelling usually involves relating the time and place, strengthening the whole record, as well as thinking about and organising the memory for the event, improving the integration of the representation into the system as a whole. Some researchers also believe that one purpose of dreams is to repeat important memories through the cortical networks to strengthen memory traces.[24]

The emotional impact of an event is also important. If strong emotions are evoked by an event, part of the emotional response is to flood the declarative memory system with neurotransmitters that boost the strength of the resulting impression left within its networks.[25] This is the basis of so-called 'flashbulb memories'.[26] The shock of some events (e.g. hearing of the death of Princess Diana) permits for an enduring and vivid recollection of the time and place where the event occurred.

A significant majority of experiences, however, are generic and mundane in nature. The memory representations that form around events that occur regularly extract the core, common aspects, but the incidental detail, which includes the time and place of learning, decays away or becomes confused with subsequent and similar experiences.[22] For example, if someone asks you whether you locked the door this morning it is very difficult to remember the specific act of locking it today, as opposed to yesterday, or the day before that, and the day before that … Thus, the majority of information in the long-term archives is semantic in nature; useful knowledge that is not tied to the time and place of learning. Most semantic knowledge becomes organised into 'schemata', mental representations that pool experiences to generate frameworks about common situations or events that aid comprehension[26] and guide behaviour.[27] The example above refers to the schema for locking the door. Also within the knowledge stores will be schema for eating at a restaurant, getting ready for bed, taking the children to school and all manner of other regular human activities. Naturally, however, the type of schemata stored and the strength of representation will depend upon a person's culture and individual life history. If a person gets Alzheimer's disease it is possible to predict their declarative memory system will deteriorate, but without knowledge of that person's life it is very difficult to know the contents of that memory system, and hence to predict how damage is likely to affect them.

This is important because memory is a far more active psychological process than is generally thought. Metaphors of memory as a box of photographs or a library highlight the passive storage aspects of memory. However, the contents of the memory archives are in constant use because one key function of memory is to make sense of the here and now. Look at Figure 12.2 – is it a rabbit or a duck? In this illusion the same picture can activate alternative concepts within semantic memory. Thus, there is a choice about how to perceive it, depending upon which interpretation is mapped onto the picture.

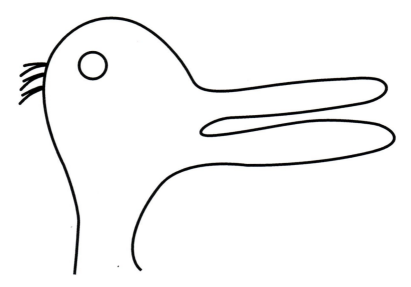

Figure 12.2 What do you see? An illustration of how concepts stored in memory influence perception

To aid this interpretative function of the memory archives, the perception of people, places or objects in the current environment automatically stimulates related memories within the declarative memory system (see Groeger[14] for a review). You may have had the experience of returning to an old childhood haunt to find that all sorts of memories come flooding back that you have not thought about for many years. It is also known that once related memories are activated, there are processes that 'smooth' over any holes in the records to form a coherent interpretation. Cleverly designed experiments can reliably trick people into remembering things that are very plausible but that did not actually happen.[28]

Perception of people, places and objects has the same effect on people with Alzheimer's disease; related memories in the archives are activated by what they see in the here and now. However, because of the damage described above, the range of information available has become restricted and the holes in the records have become bigger. But, as with normal subjects, the system continues to 'fill them in' by drawing on the available information. Together, these principles can explain many of the misperceptions and misbeliefs commonly experienced by people with Alzheimer's disease.

The effects of Alzheimer's disease are such that recent memories are subject to what could be called a 'double whammy'. Early damage to the hippocampus means that ongoing experiences are no longer captured for future reference. For the person, therefore, it is as if most things from the past few years never happened and, because the hippocampus is the gateway to the long-term archives, the archives also start to 'go out of date'. This phenomenon is exacerbated when the pathology spreads out to affect the archives themselves through damage to the cortex of the temporal lobe. The influence of age of acquisition in strengthening a memory means that as the disease process slowly but relentlessly pulls brain cells out of the archiving networks, memories are lost according to a 'last in, first out' principle.[20]

Imagine, therefore, that my grandmother has Alzheimer's disease and my brother comes to pay her a visit. If a picture of my 60-year-old father is placed next to my 30-year-old brother the family resemblance is hard to see because of the age difference. But when a photograph of my 30-year-old father is placed next to my 30-year-old brother the similarity is much more striking. Within my grandmother's mental archives, recent memories about my brother are likely to have been lost, whilst those about my father in his younger days are likely to remain. As the disease advances, therefore, it becomes increasingly likely that my grandmother interprets my 30-year-old brother to be my 30-year-old father.

Furthermore, because strong memories relate to the frequently done rather than to the rarely done, a person's past has a strong influence on which particular sets of schemata are most strongly represented within the long-term archives, as noted earlier. Schemata are powerful because they are not merely passive bundles of knowledge, but frameworks within which environments are actively understood and expectations about behaviour are generated.[27] For people who have spent much of their adult life bringing up children, schemata relating to collecting from school, preparing dinner and the bedtime routine will be particularly strong. The sight or sound of children may activate memories about being a mother, which in turn generates a belief that certain actions relating to the care of children are necessary. For a retired teacher, the sight of a room full of tables and chairs may be interpreted as a classroom rather than a dining room; for a farmer, early mornings may stimulate the schema about feeding animals; for the travelling executive, the fading light may stimulate the schema related to finding a hotel for the night.

Overall, there is increasing likelihood that the consciousness of the person is filled with memories from the past, and that the ability to distinguish between past and present deteriorates to the extent that now is literally interpreted as being then. It is important to recognise that for the person with Alzheimer's disease their conviction in their belief is as strong as if it were true. Failure to acknowledge the beliefs of people with dementia can all too easily lead to unnecessary conflict and distress.

Imagine a woman is at home. She has just had lunch and is busy tidying up the kitchen. She believes that when she has finished tidying up she must go and fetch her children from school. This is a powerful belief that must be acted on. If, in reality, someone came into her home and prevented her from fetching her children she would become agitated. If that person continued to impede her, she would become increasingly distressed and may even resort to physical violence in order to get rid of the person. If this really happened most people would be forgiving about her aggressive act because they would see the unreasonableness of a person trying to stop a mother from collecting her children from school.

But now imagine that same woman is living in a care home because she has Alzheimer's disease. She has just finished lunch and everything is being tidied up. She tries to find her coat and leave to fetch her children. But her coat is missing and the staff will not let her out of the building. In her panic she screams and lashes out at the member of staff. In this situation the woman's behaviour is less likely to be forgiven because, from the point of view of observers, her behaviour is unprovoked and unreasonable. It is only when the effects of the neurological impairment are taken into account that the important similarity between her behaviour and that of a mother dealing with an intruder who is preventing her from fetching her children becomes apparent.

This brings us back to Kitwood's model of dementia[4] in which neurological impairment plays a role, but interacts with psychological and social factors. Neurological impairment has contributed to the situation described above. Loss of cells from the declarative memory system has caused the woman to form the false belief that she is a mother who needs to collect her child from school. However, her past life and psychology are still retained within the damaged memory system, and her state of mind cannot be understood without reference to her life history. Furthermore, the act of aggression is not directly caused by this neurological impairment. It is the behaviour of other people in response to her belief that is the trigger. If someone had reassured her that her child is safe, it is unlikely she would have become so distressed and ultimately aggressive.

UNDERSTANDING BEHAVIOUR

It is hoped that the content of this chapter illustrates how the understanding of brain function that has emerged from neuropsychology underpins rather than conflicts with a person-centred approach to dementia care. The neurological element has a difficult history within the understanding of behaviour in dementia. As noted at the outset, the presence of neurological impairment has been applied in an overly narrow way to deflect attention away from the influence of powerful psychological and social factors. There is a growing evidence base to support Kitwood's contention that psychological and social factors influence behaviour.[4] Comprehensive, individualised assessments of behaviours, followed by tailored alterations to psychological or social factors, can produce significant reductions in the occurrence of those behaviours.[29,30]

Research also shows that training staff to understand the principles of person-centred care reduces the use of antipsychotic drugs.[31] There is no doubt, therefore, that the neurological element must not be used in isolation.

However, when it comes to education about dementia, it is important that the neurological element is not neglected. Education about the brain and behaviour in dementia care can promote acceptance and tolerance with regard to some forms of difficult behaviour because people come to understand that the behaviour is beyond the person's control.[32] In the past, clinicopathological research has not been especially fine grained with respect to understanding relations between brain damage and clinical consequence. Global measures, such as the Neuropsychiatric Inventory[33] (NPI) or the concept of Behavioural and Psychological Symptoms of Dementia[34] (BPSD), are often used, even though the neural underpinnings of the different behaviours rated or grouped together are very different. More recent research, however, is applying advances in technology and understanding to perform more detailed studies looking at the neuropathological correlates of specific behaviours.[35,36] It is hoped that this new knowledge will lead to methods, for example, through neuroimaging, whereby the neurological element could be more accurately assessed, helping carers to identify the situations in which psychological and social interventions are most likely to be successful. The possibility that there may be instances in which neurological damage is the prime cause, and social and psychological factors are of limited value in explaining the behaviour, needs to be held in mind because in such a situation carers need to be reassured that it is not 'their fault' that an intervention has failed despite all their best efforts.

Acknowledging that there may be situations in which behaviour is driven primarily by neurological damage is not the same as saying that a person with dementia should be reduced to 'a brain on legs' and no longer treated with dignity and respect. An aspect of brain damage often overlooked in dementia is that the damaged brain continues to be active and to operate according to the same principles as the healthy brain, albeit at a lower level. The behaviours (of people without dementia) associated with Kitwood's Malignant Social Psychology (e.g. objectification, invalidation, intimidation, ignoring[4]) are associated with a negative body language which will be picked up and processed by structures deep in the brain that are less likely to be damaged in most forms of dementia. Thus, contrary to popular belief, people with dementia do know when they are being treated dismissively, and this has the normal impact, generating defensive behaviours around fight, flight, agitation or withdrawal. It is not surprising, therefore, that poor care environments are associated with high levels of distressed behaviour.[37]

Cheston and Bender[38] note that a service implication of the organic model of dementia is that it 'encourages, rather than provides scientific evidence for, therapeutic nihilism' (p. 76). The available evidence, however, overwhelmingly shows that the prime causes of dementia are organic in nature. Progress in dementia care requires that the organic basis of the condition be accepted without a collapse into therapeutic nihilism. It is hoped that the illustration provided by this chapter shows that this is possible. Now that knowledge about the brain and its many functions is advancing it should be possible for the neurological to be more effectively integrated with the psychological and social when it comes to understanding not just dementia, but the person with dementia.

Key points

➤ An accurate understanding of behavioural change in dementia requires good knowledge of the neurology of the causes of dementia and the impact on brain function.

➤ However, because behaviour is specific to an individual and their environmental context, the neurological damage must be assessed within a framework that also takes account of psychological and social influences.

➤ This is illustrated with respect to the impact of Alzheimer's disease on the memory systems of the brain, which are centred in the temporal lobes.

➤ The nature of the pathology and the organisation of information within the temporal lobes means that the recent past suffers a 'double whammy' and the consciousness of the person is increasingly dominated by remote rather than recent events.

➤ As the disease progresses it is increasingly probable that events occurring now are interpreted in terms of things that happened long ago and, because memories provide the framework around which we organise our behaviour, behaviour is increasingly driven by outdated information.

➤ Many behaviours that seem at first sight to be unreasonable (e.g. becoming aggressive with a member of staff who is trying to protect the person by preventing them from leaving the building) are understandable and natural from within the person's outdated reality (e.g. becoming aggressive with someone who is preventing you from collecting your child from school).

➤ To understand the behaviour of a person with Alzheimer's disease, therefore, it is necessary to understand all of the following: the impact of the pathology, the person's life history and the reactions of other people to the person's confusion.

REFERENCES

1 Snowden JS, Neary D, Mann DMA. *Fronto-Temporal Lobar Degeneration, Progressive Aphasia and Semantic Dementia*. Edinburgh: Churchill Livingstone; 1996.

2 Massimo L, Powers C, Moore P, *et al.* Neuroanatomy of apathy and disinhibition in frontotemporal lobar degeneration. *Dementia Geriatr Cogn Dis.* 2009; **27**(1): 96–104.

3 Palmer AM, Stratmann GC, Procter AW, *et al.* Possible neurotransmitter basis of behavioural changes in Alzheimer's disease. *Ann Neurol.* 1988; **23**: 616–20.

4 Kitwood T. *Dementia Reconsidered.* Buckingham: Open University Press; 1997.

5 Jellinger KA. Clinicopathological analysis of dementia disorders in the elderly – an update. *J Alz Dis.* 2006; **9**(Suppl. 3): 61–70.

6 Van Hoesen GW, Damasio AR. Neural correlates of cognitive impairment in Alzheimer's disease. In: Mountcastle VB, Plum F, Oeiger SR (eds). *The Handbook of Physiology, Volume 5.* Bethesda, MD: American Physiological Society; 1987.

7 Braak H, Braak E. Neuropathological staging of Alzheimer-related changes. *Acta Neuropath (Berl).* 1991; **82**: 239–59.

8 Scoville WB, Milner B. Loss of recent memory after bilateral hippocampal lesions. *J Neurol Neurosurg Psychiat.* 1957; **20**: 11–21.

9 Kolb B, Whishaw IQ. *Fundamentals of Human Neuropsychology.* 6th ed. New York: Worth Publishers; 2003.

10 Perrin T, May H, Anderson E. *Wellbeing in Dementia: an occupational approach for therapists and carers.* Edinburgh: Churchill Livingstone, Elsevier; 2008.

11 Cohen NJ. Preserved learning capacity in amnesia: evidence for multiple memory systems. In: Squires LR, Butters N (eds). *Neuropsychology of Memory.* New York: Guildford Press; 1984. pp. 83–103.

12 Tulving E. Episodic and semantic memory. In: Tulving E, Donaldson W (eds). *Organisation of Memory.* New York: Academic Press; 1972.

13 McClelland JL, McNaughton BL, O'Reilly RC. Why are there complementary learning systems in the hippocampus and neocortex: insights from the successes and failures of connectionist models of learning and memory. *Psych Rev.* 1995; **102**(3): 419–57.

14 Groeger JA. *Memory and Remembering: everyday memory in context.* Harlow, Essex: Addison Wesley Longman Ltd; 1997.

15 Damasio AR, Damasio H, Tranel D, *et al.* Neural regionalization of knowledge access: preliminary evidence. *Symposia on Quantitative Biology.* 1990; **55**: 1039–47.

16 MacKinnon D, Squire LR. Autobiographical memory and amnesia. *Psychobiol.* 1989; **17**: 247–56.

17 Squire LR. Memory and the hippocampus: a synthesis from findings with rats, monkeys and humans. *Psych Rev.* 1992; **99**(2):195–231.

18 Fritzen J. Intralist repetition effects in free recall. *J Exp Psychol: Hum Learn Mem.* 1975; **104**: 756–63.

19 Carroll JB, White MN. Word frequency and age of acquisition as determiners of picture naming latency. *Quart J Exp Psychol.* 1973, **12**: 85–95.

20 Ellis AW, Venneri A, Shanks MF. Words, dementia and the brain. *Biologist.* 2006; **53**(3): 124–8.

21 Craik FIM, Lockhart RS. Levels of processing: a framework for memory research. *J Verb Learn Verb Behav.* 1972; **11**: 671–84.

22 Trafimow D, Wyer RS. Cognitive representation of mundane social events. *J Personality Soc Psychol.* 1993; **64**: 365–76.

23 Damasio AR. Timelocked multiregional retroactivation: a systems-level proposal for the neural substrates of recall and recognition. *Cogn.* 1989; **33**: 25–62.

24 Stickgold R. Sleep: off-line memory reprocessing. *Trends Cogn Sci.*1998; **2**(12): 484–92.

25 Cahill L, Babinsky R, Moscovitch HJ, *et al.* The amygdala and emotional memory. *Nature.* 1995; **377**: 295–6.

26 Bartlett FC. *Remembering.* Cambridge: Cambridge University Press; 1932.

27 Belson RP. Psychological status of the script concept. *Am Psychologist.* 1981; **36**: 715–29.

28 Loftus EF. Creating false memories. In: The Editors of Scientific American (eds). *The Scientific American Book of the Brain.* Guilford, CT: The Lyons Press; 1999. pp. 119–27.

29 Moniz-Cook E, Stokes G, Agar S. Difficult behaviour and dementia in nursing homes: five cases of psychosocial intervention. *Clin Psychol Psychother.* 2003; **10**: 197–208.

30 James I, Mackenzie L, Stephenson M, *et al.* Dealing with challenging behaviour through and analysis of need: the Colombo approach. In: Marshall M, Allen K (eds). *Dementia: walking not wandering.* London: Hawker; 2006.

31 Fossey J, Ballard C, Juszczak E, *et al.* Effect of enhanced psychosocial care on antipsychotic use in nursing home residents with severe dementia: cluster randomized trial. *BMJ.* 2006; **332**: 756–61.

32 Milwain E. The brain and person-centred care: bringing different perspectives together. *Journal of Dementia Care.* 2009; Nov/Dec: 22–4.

33 Cummings JL, Mega M, Gray K, *et al.* The Neuropsychiatric Inventory: comprehensive assessment of psychopathology in dementia. *Neurol.* 1994; **44**(12): 2308–14.

34 Finkel SI, Costa e Silva J, Cohen GD, *et al.* Behavioural and psychological symptoms of dementia: a consensus statement on current knowledge and implications for research and treatment. *Am J Geriatr Psychiat.* 1998; **6**(2): 97–100.

35 Apostolova LG, Akopyan GG, Partiali N, *et al.* Structural correlates of apathy in Alzheimer's disease. *Dementia Geriatr Cog Dis.* 2007; **24**(2): 91–7.

36 Nelson RJ, Trainor BC. Neural correlates of aggression. *Nature Rev: Neurosci.* 2007; **8**(7): 536–46.

37 Cohen-Mansfield J. Nonpharmacological interventions for persons with dementia. *Alz Care Quart.* 2005; **6**(2): 129–45.

38 Cheston R, Bender M. *Understanding Dementia: the man with worried eyes.* London: Jessica Kingsley Publishers; 2003.

CHAPTER 13

Legal aspects of management

Shabir Musa, Arun Devasahayam and
Jayanthi Devi Subramani

INTRODUCTION

This chapter has been written with detailed reference to the law in England and Wales. Though details are different in different jurisdictions, the same principles apply. People suffering from dementia exhibit various clinical features, including decline in cognition, intellectual functioning, reasoning ability, judgement and insight. Several legal issues arise in relation to the management of people with dementia. Capacity is the central issue in many cases. The Mental Capacity Act 2005, Mental Health Act 1983 and Deprivation of Liberty Safeguards provide us with statutory principles and framework which help, support and protect people suffering from dementia and their carers.

CAPACITY

Capacity is the 'ability to make a decision'. Capacity is a legal concept and it is defined in personal law (the part of law that deals with the matters pertaining to a person and his or her family) as 'a status' which determines whether they may make binding amendments to their rights, duties, obligations, such as getting married, entering into contracts, making gifts and writing a valid will. For the purpose of the Mental Capacity Act, a person lacks capacity in relation to a matter if, at the material time, he or she is unable to make a decision or communicate the decision because of an impairment of, or a disturbance in the functioning of, the mind or brain.[1]

In English law, an adult has the right to make decisions affecting his or her own life, whether the reasons for the choice are rational, irrational, unknown or even non-existent. This right remains even if the outcome of the decision might be detrimental to the individual. However, such a right to self-determination is meaningful only if the individual is appropriately informed, has the ability (capacity) to make the decision and is free to decide without coercion.[2] An adult is presumed to have the capacity until the contrary is proven, and a person who legally lacks capacity remains in that state until the contrary is proven.

Medical practitioners are frequently asked to give opinions about individuals' capacity. Psychiatrists are usually consulted about capacity issues in complex cases, and when someone is suspected of, or is, suffering from a mental disorder such as dementia. In disputed cases of capacity, the courts make the final decision.

MENTAL CAPACITY ACT 2005

The Mental Capacity Act 2005 for England and Wales received Royal Assent on 7 April 2005 and came into force in October 2007. The Act affects people aged 16 or over and provides a statutory framework to empower and protect people who may lack capacity to make some decisions for themselves.[3] The Act covers a wide range of decisions made, or actions taken, on behalf of people lacking capacity. These can be decisions about day-to-day matters, such as what to wear, what to buy when doing the weekly shopping, or decisions about major life-changing events such as whether the person should move into a care home or undergo a major surgical operation. The Act also stipulates decisions which cannot be made by others even though a person lacks capacity. Some of these decisions are concerning family relationships such as consenting to marriage or civil partnership, sexual relationship, divorce or dissolution of a civil partnership. Other decisions include voting rights, unlawful killing and assisted suicide.

The Mental Capacity Act is underpinned by five statutory principles (*see* Box 13.1). These are intended to support, protect and assist people who may lack capacity to make particular decisions. They are not intended to restrict or control these people's lives. When the principles are followed and applied to the decision-making framework, they will help people to take appropriate actions in individual cases. The principles are also intended to help people to find the right solutions in difficult and uncertain situations.

ASSESSMENT OF CAPACITY

To help determine one's ability to make decisions, the Mental Capacity Act sets out a two-stage test to assess capacity.

Stage 1

Does the person have an impairment of the mind or brain, or is there some sort of disturbance affecting the way their mind or brain works? (It does not matter whether the impairment or disturbance is temporary or permanent.)

Box 13.1   Mental Capacity Act 2005: five statutory principles

1   A person must be assumed to have capacity unless it is established that he lacks capacity.
2   A person is not to be treated as unable to make a decision unless all practicable steps to help him to do so have been taken without success.
3   A person is not to be treated as unable to make a decision merely because he makes an unwise decision.
4   An act done, or decision made, under this Act for or on behalf of a person who lacks capacity must be done, or made, in his best interests.
5   Before the act is done, or the decision is made, regard must be had to whether the purpose for which it is needed can be as effectively achieved in a way that is less restrictive of the person's rights and freedom of action.

Stage 2

If so, does that impairment or disturbance mean that the person is unable to make the decision in question at the time it needs to be made?

A person is unable to make a decision if they cannot meet the criteria listed in Box 13.2.

Box 13.2   Definition of 'Inability to make a decision'

A person in unable to make a decision if they cannot:
➤   understand information about the decision to be made
➤   retain that information in their mind
➤   use or weigh that information as part of the decision-making process or
➤   communicate their decision (by talking, using sign language or any other means).

Special efforts should be made when assessing capacity of a person with cognitive impairment. Before the assessment, it is helpful to collect background information about the person. The presence of a friend or relative might make the person feel at ease and might help them understand the information. However, their right to confidentiality should be respected. Relevant information should be provided in a simple and clear fashion. Too much information might confuse them. The time of the day and place where the assessment takes place might help them in decision making. The information may need to be repeated many times in some situations. Enough time should be given for the person to arrive at their decision. For persons with communication difficulties, every effort should be made to find alternative ways to help them in the decision-making process. For example, interpreters, sign language specialists, pictures and written materials should be used as appropriate.

BEST INTERESTS

Many different people may be required to make decisions or act on behalf of a person who lacks capacity to make decisions for themselves. Under the Act, they are referred as 'decision-maker'. Depending upon the situation they could be nurses, doctors, carers, attorneys or deputies appointed by Court of Protection. The Act requires the decision-makers to make decisions in the best interest of the person who lacks capacity. As a matter of good practice it is advisable to obtain a second opinion from another doctor in cases where a complex decision is contemplated.

When arriving at the person's best interests, consideration should be given to the:
➤ past and present wishes of the person
➤ need to maximise the person's participation in the decision
➤ views of others as to the person's wishes and feelings and
➤ need to adopt the course of action that is least restrictive to the person's freedom.

There are two circumstances when the best interests principle will not apply. The first is where someone has previously made an advance decision to refuse medical treatment while they had the capacity to do so. Their advance decision should be respected when they lack capacity, even if others think that the decision to refuse treatment is not in their best interests. The second one is participation in research when they lack capacity to consent.

POWERS OF ATTORNEY

A power of attorney is a deed by which one person (the 'donor') gives another person (the 'attorney') the authority to act in the donor's name and on his or her behalf. It is possible to choose more than one attorney. If more than one attorney is chosen, then they could act either jointly (that is, they must all act together and cannot act separately) or jointly and severally (that is, they can all act together but they can also act separately if they wish).

There are two types of powers of attorney, ordinary power of attorney and lasting power of attorney.

Ordinary power of attorney

Ordinary powers of attorney are created for a set period of time in cases where the donor is going abroad or is unable to act for some other reason and wishes someone else to have the authority to act on his or her behalf. The ordinary power of attorney can be specific or general. If it is specific, the attorney only has the authority to do the things specified by the donor in the power. If it is general, the attorney has the authority to do anything that the donor can lawfully do with his or her property and affairs.

The test of capacity, which a person must satisfy in order to make an ordinary power of attorney, is that the donor understands the nature and effect of what he or she is doing. Although the legal form completed by the donor is usually simple, it is generally advisable to seek legal advice. There is no requirement to register the ordinary power of attorney. An ordinary power of attorney ceases to have effect if the donor becomes mentally incapable, for example, if they develop significant dementia. The donor or the attorney can cancel the ordinary power of attorney at any time.

Lasting power of attorney

The lasting power of attorney (LPA) replaced the enduring power of attorney (EPA) from October 2007. There are two types of LPA: personal welfare LPA and property and affairs LPA. The Mental Capacity Act stipulates what the LPAs are and how they should be used.

Procedure

The donor must follow the right procedures for creating and registering the LPA for it to be valid. They can only make a LPA if they have the 'capacity' to do so. There are separate statutory forms for the personal welfare LPA and the property and affairs LPA.

For a LPA to be valid the following conditions musts be met.

➤ The donor must sign a statement confirming that they have read the prescribed information (or somebody has read it to them).

➤ The document should state the names of people (not any of the attorneys) who should be notified when an application to register the LPA is being made. However, the donor could choose not to name anyone to be notified.

➤ The attorneys must sign a statement saying that they have read the prescribed information and that they understand their duties, in particular the duty to act in the donor's best interests.

➤ The document must include a certificate completed by an independent person certifying that in their opinion, at the time the LPA is made:

   – the donor understands the purpose of the LPA and scope of the authority under it

- no fraud or undue pressure is being used to induce the donor to create the LPA and
- there is nothing else that would prevent the LPA being created.

The LPA must be registered with the Office of the Public Guardian (OPG) before it can be used. The donor can register the LPA when they are still capable and the attorney can register it at any time. All EPAs which were in existence in October 2007 must be registered with the OPG for them to be valid.

Personal welfare LPA

The personal welfare LPA allows someone to choose one or more people to make decisions on their behalf with regards to their personal welfare and healthcare. This includes consenting or refusing medical treatments and decisions about where to live. If the donor wants the attorney to make decisions about life-sustaining treatment, they should express this specifically on the form. The attorney cannot consent on behalf of the donor about a treatment for which the donor has made an advance decision. The attorney of a personal welfare LPA cannot make decisions about property and financial affairs.

Property and affairs LPA

The property and affairs LPA allows someone to choose one or more people to make decisions about their property and affairs (including financial matters). If there are no restrictions stipulated on the LPA, the attorney(s) can make any decisions about the finances, such as buying or selling property, operating bank accounts, managing investments, receiving income, inheritance and any entitlement on behalf of the donor.

Court appointed deputy

The Mental Capacity Act 2005 provides for a system of court appointed deputies to replace the old system of receivership. Deputies will be able to take decisions on welfare, healthcare and financial matters as authorised by the Court of Protection. The Court of Protection will not give authority to the deputies to make decisions about life-sustaining treatment. They will only be appointed if the Court cannot make a one-off decision to resolve the issues and no valid LPA is in place. Usually deputies are necessary when a series of decisions need to be made regarding property and financial affairs. If the only income of a person who lacks capacity is social security benefits and they have no property or savings, there will usually be no need for a deputy to be appointed. This is because the person's benefits can be managed by an *appointee*, appointed by the Department for Work and Pensions to receive and deal with the benefits of a person who lacks capacity to do this for themselves. Deputies for personal welfare are needed in situations when someone has to make a series of welfare decisions over time and it would not be beneficial or appropriate to require all these decisions to be made by the court; or there is a history of serious family disputes that could have a detrimental effect on the person's future care unless a deputy is appointed to make necessary decisions.

APPOINTEESHIP

The appointeeship system enables another individual, known as an appointee, to receive and administer social security benefits and allowances on behalf of a mentally incapable person. Appointeeship is governed by regulation 33 of the Social Security (Claims and Payments) Regulations 1987. Medical evidence of the claimant's inability to manage his or her own affairs may be requested.

The Secretary of State can revoke an appointment at any time, and there is no right of appeal to a tribunal against the Secretary of State's refusal to appoint a particular individual as appointee or against the revocation of such an appointment. Appointees have no authority to deal with the claimant's capital. If the Court of Protection appoints a deputy to manage property and affairs, it is likely that the deputy will take over the appointee's role.

INDEPENDENT MENTAL CAPACITY ADVOCATE (IMCA)

An IMCA is someone appointed by the local authority or NHS organisation to support a person who lacks capacity and there is no one to speak on their behalf, such as family or friends. IMCAs are involved when decisions are being made about serious medical treatment, when deprivation of liberty is being considered or when a change in the person's accommodation to the one provided by the NHS or a local authority is proposed. They are also to be involved whenever a person who lacks capacity with no unpaid carers remains in hospital for more than 28 days or in a care home for more than eight weeks. The IMCA makes representations about the person's wishes, feelings, beliefs and values, at the same time as bringing to the attention of the decision-maker all factors that are relevant to the decision. The IMCA can challenge the decision-maker on behalf of the person lacking capacity, if necessary.

ADVANCE DECISIONS

If an individual is found to lack capacity, then reference should be made to any advance decisions the person may have made. The Mental Capacity Act sets out guidance when someone has made an advance decision to refuse treatment. Advance decisions are declarations whereby competent people make known their views on what should happen if they lose the capacity to make decisions for themselves. This allows people to state which treatments they would or would not want if they become seriously ill and no longer have the mental capacity to make decisions. Advance decisions can take a variety of forms, ranging from general lists of life values and preferences to specific requests or refusals. They can be written or oral. Advance decisions about refusing life-sustaining treatments should be written, signed and witnessed. They should also clearly state that the decision applies even when the life is at risk.

The test for capacity to make an advance statement about medical treatment is similar to that for capacity to make a contemporaneous medical decision. In order for an advance statement to be valid the patient must have been competent when the statement was made, must have been acting free from pressure and must have been offered sufficient, accurate information to make an informed decision. It is recommended that advance statements be updated regularly, usually every three years, to indicate that they truly reflect the person's current views.

OFFICE OF THE PUBLIC GUARDIAN

The Public Guardian has several duties under the Act and is supported in carrying these out by an OPG. The OPG registers LPAs and the EPAs. It also supervises the deputies appointed by the Court of Protection and provides information to help the Court make decisions. The OPG is an agency of the Ministry of Justice and works with other agencies, such as the police and social services, to respond to any concerns raised about the way in which an attorney or deputy is operating. A Public Guardian Board scrutinises and reviews the way in which the OPG discharges its functions.

COURT OF PROTECTION

The Mental Capacity Act provided for a new Court of Protection to make decisions in relation to 'property and affairs' and 'health and welfare' of someone who lacks capacity. It also has power to make declarations about whether someone has the capacity to make a particular decision. The Court has the same powers, rights, privileges and authority in relation to mental capacity matters as the High Court. It is a superior court of record and is able to set precedents.

The Court of Protection has the powers to:

➤ decide whether a person has capacity to make a particular decision
➤ make declarations, decisions or orders on financial or welfare matters affecting people who lack capacity
➤ appoint deputies to make decisions for people lacking capacity
➤ Decide whether a LPA or EPA is valid
➤ make decisions on cases concerning objections to register a LPA or EPA
➤ remove deputies or attorneys who fail to carry out their duties
➤ make decisions on cases relevant to Deprivation of Liberty Safeguards
➤ decide whether an advance decision is valid.

CAPACITY TO MAKE A WILL

A will is a document in which the maker (called the 'testator' if he is a man and the 'testatrix' if she is a woman) appoints an executor to deal with their affairs when they die and describes how their estate is to be distributed after their death.[4] The degree of understanding, which the law requires a person making a will to have, is known as *testamentary capacity*. Testamentary capacity should be present both when giving instructions for the preparation of the will and at the time of execution or signing of the will. A greater degree of mental capacity is likely to be required when making a complex will in comparison to a simple will.

The criteria listed in Box 13.3 should be assessed in deciding whether an individual has testamentary capacity.

Box 13.3   Testamentary capacity

An individual making a will should:
➤ understand the nature of the act and its effects
➤ understand the nature and extent of the property being disposed
➤ be able to distinguish and compare potential beneficiaries
➤ be free from an abnormal state of mind.

A person with mental disorder may legitimately make a will, provided the mental disorder does not influence any of the criteria relevant to the making of the will. Old age psychiatrists and GPs are most likely to be asked to give their opinion as to testamentary capacity in cases of presumed or established dementia. Solicitors are advised that when drawing up a will for an elderly person or someone who is seriously ill, they should ensure the will is witnessed or approved by a medical practitioner. The medical practitioner should record his or her examination and findings. The capacity to revoke a will is the same as the capacity to make a will in the first place. A will is automatically revoked when the person gets married.

Statutory wills

If a person is both (a) incapable, by reason of mental disorder, of managing and administering his or her property and affairs and (b) incapable of making a valid will, an application can be made to the Court of Protection for a statutory will to be drawn up and executed on the person's behalf. The Court requires medical evidence of both types of incapacity. The Court is obliged to make a will, consistent with the one the patient would have made for him- or herself, within reason, and with competent legal advice.

MENTAL HEALTH ACT 1983

In 2007, several amendments were made to the Mental Health Act 1983 (MHA). Patients with dementia may become subject to various sections of the MHA.[5] For a detailed account of all the possible sections of the MHA that are applicable to patients with dementia, the reader is referred to the *Mental Health Act Manual*.[6] A brief account of the commonly applied sections of the MHA relevant to people with dementia is provided below.

Section 5(2): Doctor's holding power

An informal in-patient who wishes to leave hospital may be detained for up to 72 hours if the doctor believes an application should be made for compulsory admission under the MHA. This requires a single medical recommendation by the doctor in charge of the patient's care, or his or her nominated deputy. It is usual to consider a change to a section 2 or 3 order as soon as possible.[7]

Section 2: Assessment order

Criteria

Section 2 provides that a person may be detained under the MHA for a period of up to 28 days on the grounds that the person:

➤ is suffering from a mental disorder of a nature or degree which warrants their detention in hospital for assessment (or for assessment followed by treatment) for at least a limited period and

➤ ought to be so detained in the interests of their own health or safety or with a view to the protection of others.

Procedure

The section 2 procedure requires the following.

➤ Application by the patient's nearest relative or an approved mental health professional (AMHP) who must have seen the patient within the last 14 days. The AMHP should, so far as it is practicable, consult the nearest relative.

➤ Medical recommendations by two doctors, one of whom must be approved under section 12 of the MHA. If the medical recommendations are performed separately, then they should be done within five days of each other.

Section 3: Treatment order

Criteria

Section 3 provides that a person may be detained under the MHA for an initial period of up to six months on the grounds that:

➤ the person is suffering from a mental disorder of a nature or degree which makes it appropriate for them to receive medical treatment in hospital

➤ it is necessary for the health or safety of the person or for the protection of other persons that they should receive such treatment and it cannot be provided unless the patient is detained under this section
➤ appropriate medical treatment is available.

Procedure

The section 3 procedure requires the following.
➤ Application by the patient's nearest relative or an AMHP. The AMHP must, if practicable, consult the nearest relative before making an application and cannot proceed if the nearest relative objects.
➤ Medical recommendations similar to those for section 2. In addition, the recommendations must state the particular grounds for the doctor's opinion, specifying whether any other methods of dealing with the patient are available and, if so, why they are not appropriate.

When making recommendations for detention under section 3, doctors are required to state that appropriate medical treatment is available for the patient. Preferably, they should know in advance of making the recommendation the name of the hospital to which the patient is to be admitted. But if that is not possible, their recommendation may state that appropriate medical treatment will be available if the patient is admitted to one or more specific hospitals (or units within a hospital). The order may be renewed on the first occasion for a further six months and subsequently for a year at a time.

Section 7: Guardianship order

The purpose of guardianship is to enable patients to receive community care where it cannot be provided without the use of compulsory powers. It provides an authoritative framework for working with a patient, with a minimum constraint, to achieve as independent a life as possible within the community.

Procedure

The application, medical recommendations, duration and renewal are similar to those for section 3 of the MHA. The guardian is usually the local social services authority. Sometimes a private individual is appointed as the guardian. The guardian has a number of powers and these are detailed in Box 13.4.

The guardian can use this power to convey the patient to the required place of residence. There is no power to force entry into the patient's home if the patient refuses access. For guardianship to be successful a degree of co-operation is required from the patient.

Box 13.4   Powers of guardianship

The guardian has three specific powers:
1   they have exclusive rights to decide where the patient should live
2   they can require the patient to attend for treatment, work, training or education at specific times and places (but they cannot use force to take the patient there)
3   they can demand that a doctor, AMHP or another relevant person has access to the patient at the place where the patient lives.

DEPRIVATION OF LIBERTY SAFEGUARDS

People who suffer from a disorder or disability of mind, such as dementia, and who lack capacity to consent to the care or treatment should be cared for in a way that does not limit their rights or freedom of action. In some cases, members of this vulnerable group need to be deprived of their liberty for either treatment or care, because it is necessary in their best interests and to protect them from any harm.

The Deprivation of Liberty Safeguards, which came into force in April 2009, provide a legal framework to authorise deprivation of liberty where this is necessary to provide care and treatment for people lacking capacity.[8] These safeguards were introduced to make the English and Welsh law compatible with the European Convention on Human Rights, and the MCA 2005 has been amended to include them. The safeguards apply to people in England and Wales who have a mental disorder and lack capacity to consent to the arrangements made for their care or treatment, but for whom receiving care or treatment in circumstances that amount to a deprivation of liberty may be necessary to protect them from harm and appears to be in their best interests.

The European Court of Human Rights (ECtHR) has drawn a distinction between the deprivation of liberty of an individual (which is unlawful, unless authorised) and restrictions on the liberty of movement of an individual. The difference between deprivation of and restriction upon liberty is merely one of degree or intensity and not one of nature or substance.[9]

The following factors, which are not exhaustive, may indicate that deprivation of liberty is taking place:
➤ restraint is used, including sedation, to admit a person to an institution where that person is resisting admission
➤ staff exercise complete and effective control over the care and movement of a person for a significant period
➤ staff exercise control over assessments, treatment, contacts and residence
➤ a decision has been taken by the institution that the person will not be

released into the care of others, or permitted to live elsewhere, unless the staff in the institution consider it appropriate

➤ a request by carers for the person to be discharged to their care is refused

➤ the person is unable to maintain social contacts because of restrictions placed on their access to other people

➤ the person loses autonomy because they are under continuous supervision and control.

Deprivation of liberty process involves two key bodies, a managing authority and a supervisory body.

Managing authority

The managing authority has responsibility for applying for authorisation of deprivation of liberty for any person who may come within the scope of the Deprivation of Liberty Safeguards. It is either the hospital trust or the manager of the care home depending upon where the relevant person is.

Supervisory body

The supervisory body is responsible for considering requests for authorisations, commissioning the required assessments and, where all the assessments agree, authorising the deprivation of liberty. Where the Deprivation of Liberty Safeguards are applied to persons in hospitals, the supervisory body is the primary care trust and for persons in care home, the supervisory body is the local authority.

There are two types of authorisation: standard and urgent. A managing authority must ask the supervisory body for a standard authorisation when it appears likely that, at some time during the next 28 days, someone will be accommodated in circumstances that amount to a deprivation of liberty. Where this is not possible, the managing authority can give an urgent authorisation and then obtain standard authorisation within seven days. This can be extended for a further seven days, by the supervisory body, in exceptional circumstances.

There are six assessments that must be conducted before a supervisory body can give an authorisation.

➤ age assessment

➤ no refusals assessment

➤ mental capacity assessment

➤ mental health assessment

➤ eligibility assessment

➤ best interests assessment.

These assessments must be completed within 21 days of a request for a standard deprivation of liberty authorisation; or when an urgent authorisation has been given, before that urgent authorisation expires.

Age assessment

This is to confirm that the relevant person is over 18 years.

No refusals assessment

This is to confirm that the Deprivation of Liberty Safeguards authorisation does not conflict with any other existing authority for decision making for that person. It can include any valid advance decisions to refuse treatment made by the relevant person and any valid decision made by the attorney of LPA or by the deputy appointed by the Court of Protection.

Mental capacity assessment

The purpose of the mental capacity assessment is to establish whether the relevant person lacks capacity to decide whether or not they should be accommodated in the relevant hospital or care home to be given care or treatment.

Mental health assessment

The purpose of the mental health assessment is to establish whether the relevant person has a mental disorder within the meaning of the MHA. This is not an assessment to determine whether the person requires mental health treatment. This assessment must be done by a Deprivation of Liberty Safeguards-trained registered medical practitioner.

Eligibility assessment

This assessment relates specifically to the relevant person's status, or potential status, under the MHA. The eligibility assessment can be done by a Deprivation of Liberty Safeguards-trained, section 12-approved doctor or the best interests assessor, who is also an AMHP.

A person is not eligible for a deprivation of liberty authorisation if they:
➤ are detained as a hospital in-patient under the MHA
➤ are subject to a guardianship order or a community treatment order under the MHA and accommodating them in a particular care home would conflict with the requirement imposed on them by their guardian or by the conditions of their community treatment order
➤ meet the criteria for an application for admission under section 2 or 3 of the MHA.

Best interests assessment

The purpose of the best interests assessment is to establish whether:
➤ it is in the best interests of the relevant person to be deprived of their liberty
➤ it is necessary for them to be deprived of their liberty in order to prevent harm to themselves and

➤ deprivation of liberty is a proportionate response to the likelihood of the relevant person suffering harm and the seriousness of that harm.

The best interests assessment may be undertaken by an AMHP, social worker, nurse, occupational therapist or chartered psychologist and they should have successfully completed the training that has been approved by the Secretary of State to be a best interests assessor.

There must be a minimum of two assessors. The mental health and the best interest assessments cannot be done by the same person.

If all the assessments conclude that the relevant person meets the requirements for authorisation, then the supervisory body can give a deprivation of liberty authorisation for up to 12 months. Deprivation of liberty should last for the shortest period possible. The best interests assessor should only recommend authorisation for as long as the relevant person is likely to meet all the qualifying requirements.

The supervisory body may attach conditions to the authorisation as recommended by the best interests assessor and may add other conditions. It is the responsibility of the supervisory body to appoint a representative for the relevant person. The representative represents and supports the relevant person in all matters relating to the Deprivation of Liberty Safeguards, including, if appropriate, triggering a review, using an organisation's complaints procedure on the person's behalf or making an application to the Court of Protection.

A standard authorisation can be reviewed at any time when it is felt that the relevant person no longer meets the criteria for deprivation of liberty. This review is carried out by the supervisory body.

DEMENTIA AND DRIVING

It is the duty of the driving licence holder or the applicant to notify the Driver and Vehicle Licensing Authority (DVLA) of any medical condition which may affect safe driving.[10] The DVLA must be notified as soon as a diagnosis of dementia is made. In early dementia when sufficient skills are retained, and progression is slow, a licence may be issued subject to annual review. A formal driving assessment may be necessary. It is extremely difficult to assess driving ability in those with dementia.

There are some circumstances in which the licence holder cannot, or will not, inform the DVLA of a significant medical condition which may affect safe driving. Under these circumstances the General Medical Council has issued clear guidelines. These are as follows.

➤ The DVLA is legally responsible for deciding if a person is medically unfit to drive. It needs to know when driving licence holders have a condition that may, now or in the future, affect their safety as a driver.

➤ Therefore, where patients have such conditions, doctors should make sure that the patients understand that the condition may impair their ability to drive. If a patient is incapable of understanding this advice, for example, because of dementia, the doctor should inform the DVLA immediately. The doctor should explain to patients that he or she has a legal duty to inform the DVLA about the condition.

➤ If patients refuse to accept the diagnosis or effect of the condition on their ability to drive, the doctor can suggest that the patients seek a second opinion. The patients should be advised not to drive until the second opinion has been obtained.

➤ If patients continue to drive when they are not fit to do so, every reasonable effort should be made to persuade them to stop. This may include telling their next of kin.

➤ If the patient continues to drive contrary to medical advice, the doctor should disclose relevant medical information immediately, in confidence, to the medical adviser at the DVLA.

➤ Before giving information to the DVLA, the doctor should inform the patient of his or her decision to do so. Once the DVLA has been informed, the doctor should also write to the patient, to confirm that a disclosure has been made.

When the DVLA is notified about any relevant medical condition, the medical adviser can take several possible courses of action. They may request more information about the patient's current state of health from the GP or hospital doctor. The patient may be requested to undergo a medical examination by a doctor appointed by the DVLA. In some circumstances, the medical adviser may require the patient to be examined by a clinical psychologist. If a decision to revoke the driving licence is taken this is communicated to the patient by letter. The individual has the legal right to appeal against the decision, but such appeals are rarely successful.

CONCLUSIONS

Various medico-legal issues arise in people suffering from dementia as it is a chronic degenerative illness. There is a progressive decline in cognition, intellectual functioning, reasoning ability, judgement and insight in these patients. Issues in relation to mental capacity occur most frequently. In such situations, the Mental Capacity Act 2005 provides a statutory framework for decisions and actions to be taken in relation to the person who lacks capacity. Deprivation of Liberty Safeguards provide a legal framework to authorise deprivation of liberty where this is necessary to provide care and treatment for people lacking capacity.

Key points

➤ Capacity is a legal concept.

➤ An adult is presumed to have capacity until the contrary is proven.

➤ Most people with early dementia are capable of giving valid consent to common medical treatments.

➤ People with dementia who lack capacity and do not show any dissent to being hospitalised or to receive treatment should be treated under Mental Capacity Act. Deprivation of Liberty Safeguards should be applied, if appropriate.

➤ Advance decisions about treatment are currently valid under the Mental Capacity Act.

➤ There are two types of LPA: 'personal welfare LPA' and 'property and affairs LPA'.

➤ The attorney for a personal welfare LPA can make decisions regarding medical treatment on behalf of the person lacking capacity.

➤ A person with mental disorder may legitimately make a will, provided the mental disorder does not influence any of the criteria relevant to making of the will.

➤ The DVLA is legally responsible for deciding a person's medical fitness to drive.

REFERENCES

1 Mental Capacity Act 2005. Available at: www.legislation.gov.uk/ukpga/2005/9/contents (accessed May 2011).

2 Grisso T. *Evaluating Competencies: forensic assessments and instruments.* New York: Plenum; 1986.

3 *Mental Capacity Act 2005 – Code of Practice.* London: The Stationery Office; 2007.

4 British Medical Association and Law Society. *Assessment of Mental Capacity: a practical guide for doctors and lawyers.* 3rd ed. London: BMA; 2010.

5 Mental Health Act 2007. Available at: www.legislation.gov.uk/ukpga/2007/12/contents (accessed May 2011).

6 Jones R. *Mental Health Act Manual.* London: Sweet & Maxwell Ltd; 2008.

7 *Mental Health Act 2007 – Code of Practice.* London: The Stationery Office; 2008.

8 *Deprivation of Liberty Safeguards – Code of Practice.* London: The Stationery Office; 2008.

9 *HL v United Kingdom* (2004) 40 EHRR 761, ECtHR.

10 Driver and Vehicle Licensing Authority. *At a Glance Guide to the Current Medical Standards of Fitness to Drive for Medical Practitioners.* Swansea: DVLA; 2009.

CHAPTER 14

Spiritual aspects of dementia

Daphne Wallace

SPIRITUALITY

Spirituality is a concept that has varied interpretations. In order to talk about spiritual aspects of dementia, I feel that it is important to start with the working definition that I shall use throughout (*see* Box 14.1). John Swinton devotes the whole of his first chapter to this issue in a book exploring the spiritual aspects of mental healthcare.[1] It is a common assumption that 'spiritual' and 'religious' are interchangeable. In care plans and assessment of needs it seems often to be seen as an optional extra. Krishna Mohan, in *Consciousness and its Transformation*,[2] comments: 'Though spirituality traditionally has been considered to be exclusively the domain of religion, it is now being conceptualised in terms that have no particular relationship to theology, and is at the same time being accepted as practically and intellectually respectable.'

Box 14.1   Definition of spirituality

Spirituality may usefully be defined thus:

Spirituality is regarded as a basic characteristic of all people, which is vital to health and well-being. It is a universal search for meaning and purpose, which is an essential part of being human.

   For those with a religious faith, their relationship with God may be one of those relationships that give meaning and purpose to their lives.

SPIRITUAL CARE

In the past, spiritual care, however understood, was considered the responsibility of the hospital chaplain, minister of religion, priest or religious leader – it was left to the 'expert'.[3]

With the change to the concept of whole-person care, there is increasing awareness that spiritual well-being is relevant and important. Attention to spiritual needs leads to a better quality of life. Meeting them is not an add-on 'icing on the cake', but an integral part of whole-person care. Recognition of the personhood of the individual is vital.

As pointed out by Kitwood: 'For the greater part of the period in which dementia has existed as a clinical category, the subjectivity of those affected has been almost totally disregarded.'[4] Despite the writing of Alison Froggatt[5] when she drew attention to this area, this was not really followed up, and if so, only with those with milder cognitive disability.

For some time concern has been expressed for those with dementia. The tendency to see people with advanced dementia as non-persons is still pervasive and, despite much work to change the situation, as a group their spiritual needs tend to be particularly neglected. Reverend Eileen Shamy, a Methodist minister from New Zealand, started a ministry for those with dementia. This was partly informed by her experience of looking after her mother with dementia for 12 years. Writing with Alison Froggatt[6] and in her own book, *More than Body, Brain and Breath*,[7] she describes this experience.

Describing the last days of her mother's 12-year journey through Alzheimer's disease she says:

> Some days she forgot who I was and some days she confused me with her younger sister... at the end, only three days before her death, out of the dull grey of memory loss and confusion she said to me, firmly and clear-eyed, 'God never forgets us. Remember that, dear!' At that moment her suffering and my weary questioning was shot through with light. The whole devastating experience began to acquire new meaning. I knew then that nothing had been lost and that in the end all would be harvest. I am now committed, and others with me, to an unmapped journey, sustained by grace and deep gut prayer. It is a journey towards holistic care for people with Alzheimer's Disease and related dementias in which the spiritual dimension of care is given as much respectful attention as the physical, emotional and social dimensions.

PERSON-CENTRED CARE

Tom Kitwood's seminal work on person-centred care for those with dementia has also altered many misperceptions of the needs of people with dementia. There are many publications from the Bradford Dementia Group of Bradford University, well represented by him in *Dementia Reconsidered*[4] and *The New Culture of Dementia Care*.[8] As he pointed out, there is an 'old' and a 'new' culture of dementia care. The 'old' is well illustrated by an account of an agency's approach to a day centre wishing to promote awareness about Alzheimer's disease. They asked for some photographs of clients for publicity purposes. Permission was sought and granted and the photographs duly taken and sent. They were rejected because they did not show the disturbed and agonised characteristics that people with dementia 'ought' to show. Stirling University Dementia Services Development Centre has also published material about the needs of elderly with dementia, including spiritual needs.

COMMUNICATION

Malcolm Goldsmith, during his time at Stirling, carried out research into communication with those with dementia, published as *Hearing the Voice of People with Dementia*.[9] John Killick has developed his skills as writer and poet to help those with dementia communicate and has produced books of 'assisted' writings,[10,11] where he writes down the things said to him in conversation when visiting as writer in residence to Westminster Health Care and the Stirling Dementia Services Development Centre. As Sue Benson, editor of *Journal of Dementia Care*, says in the foreword to the collection published as *You are Words*:[10]

> John Killick's work has made two very special contributions to the cause of good practice in dementia care. Giving time and concentrated attention to an individual, listening carefully to what they say, tells each person with dementia they are valued, that they are of interest and worth. The further step of writing down what is said powerfully underlines that statement of worth.

His work has shown that even those who are severely affected by dementia, who care staff believe to be incapable of communicating, can, with attention and confidence in the listener, communicate with great clarity and insight.

Earlier diagnosis has meant that people with dementia have been able over the last few years to write about their experience. Two striking examples worth mentioning are the books by Christine Bryden[12] and Richard Taylor.[13] Christine Bryden talks about the benefit of relationships: 'How you relate to us has a big impact on the course of the disease. You can restore our personhood, and give us a sense of being needed and valued' (p. 127). Richard Taylor (p. 148) refers to the writings of Martin Buber (1878–1965) and his concern with the transition from I-Thou to I-It relationships in our society. Taylor likens his experience of Alzheimer's disease to this transition and his fear of being regarded as a non-person. Both these authors talk about the importance of communication with others in the preservation of the personhood of the person with dementia.

THE CURRENT SITUATION

Unfortunately, despite all this valuable work, many people with dementia languish in institutions with little attention paid to their individual needs, wishes and personalities. It is vital that as well as attempts to ensure sufficient space, good food, privacy and healthcare, the needs of the individual person are not ignored. Such small things can make a vital difference to the well-being of the individual. Eileen Shamy[7] gives a telling example of simple needs not met (*see* Case Study 14.1).

Case Study 14.1

Eileen Shamy describes a sequence of events with her mother:

As an example of the deprivation this can cause I think of my mother who had always been a talented needlewoman and craftsperson. Her hands were never idle. When she went into a nursing home because she needed 24-hour care she was still crocheting. She crocheted squares for afghan quilts and her work, even then, was some of the most perfectly executed I have ever seen. She took pleasure in the colours, arranging them harmoniously and crocheting the squares together. That she found the work satisfying was obvious. It seemed to me that the fact that her hands were always busy was the reason she seldom wandered or showed any impatience with being confined to the house and garden.

One weekend when it happened that I could not visit she dropped her hook and could not find it. All that day, on and off – I was told afterwards – she picked up her work and asked for her crochet hook. No one thought it important to look for it and the weekend staff did not know that she had a spare hook in her room. She still had her work-basket in the lounge on Monday when I visited again. Immediately I noticed her still hands. I picked up the partly completed quilt and she began to cry. Why was she crying? A passing regular staff remarked, 'She hasn't crocheted all day. Weekend staff told us that she was very agitated most of Saturday and Sunday. The cook said that she had lost her crochet hook.'

I went to fetch the spare hook from her room and placed it in her hands. She looked bewildered so I took it and crocheted a few stitches. I told her that she was much, much better at this than I was. But when I placed the hook in her hand she held it awkwardly and poked it aimlessly, not even connecting it to the wool. Silently she put it down and folded her hands. She never picked it up again. It was a kind of dying. I grieved for her loss.

Why had no one thought to fetch her spare hook? If I had been well enough to visit her that weekend would she still have been crocheting? If she had dropped her soup spoon someone most certainly would have replaced that for her.

> I was right to grieve. She remained sad and restless and her little hands stiffened without the exercise. Worse, another resource for nourishing her spiritual well-being was lost to her.

In 2002, the *National Minimum Standards for Care Homes for Older People*, which formed the basis on which the National Care Standards Commission inspected and regulated homes, was published.[14] It only mentions spiritual needs in the context of dying and death (Standard 11). Much work has been done by Tom Kitwood, with the Bradford University Dementia Group continuing since his death, Stirling University Dementia Services Development Centre, the Alzheimer's Society and a number of Christian organisations, including the Christian Council on Ageing (CCOA) Dementia Group, Methodist Homes, Caritas Social Action Network (that has produced an excellent DVD called *Its still ME, Lord* …)[15] and Faith in Elderly People, Leeds. All these groups have produced good material for training and increasing awareness. As Alison Johnson[16] pointed out, there is a need for sensitive care with recognition that people with dementia retain their personhood and that those with failing mental powers need in every way to be treated as persons, just as we all would like to be treated. The spiritual needs of those with dementia are not only important in institutional care. Many old people live in the community, and half of those over 75 live alone.[17]

Relatives may also fail to understand their dear ones' spiritual needs. Person-centred care can just as easily be applied at home and usually is but, importantly, good care in a residential home should not be hampered by relatives (*see* Case Studies 14.2 and 14.3).

Case Study 14.2

A retired nurse lived in a residential home. Putting on her make-up first thing in the day had always been an important part of her routine.

One day her daughter visited and her make-up was less perfectly put on than usual. With a comment that her mother was no longer capable of doing it properly, she took away all her mother's make-up items. For two or three days the resident searched for her make-up, becoming increasingly upset and agitated. Eventually the staff bought her some replacement items and she was pleased to resume her daily routine.

The daughter presumably could not cope with the lessening of competence in her mother.

Case Study 14.3

An elderly patient in a hospital continuing care ward had a number of family photographs near his bed. One day the relatives removed them all. Eventually, on enquiry, the staff discovered that they had been worried about the danger of the glass in the frames.

Unfortunately they therefore removed his special personal effects and his one contact with his family when they were not actually visiting.

SPIRITUAL CARE: MEDICAL

Psychiatrists have had problems with spiritual aspects of care. David Crossley, in an editorial in the *British Journal of Psychiatry*,[18] says: 'It comes as a surprise that psychiatrists should be so reticent in their inquiry into this aspect of their patients' emotional and cognitive experience.' Since his editorial and the earlier comments by Andrew Sims,[19] the Spirituality Interest Group in the Royal College has been founded and grown significantly in membership. As I have outlined earlier, religious belief is only one expression of the spirituality of the person.

Scott Peck[20] alludes to the criticism of atheist friends that 'religion is a crutch for old people as they face the mystery, the terror of their death'. Later in the same book he talks about: 'Our unique human capacity for change and transformation is reflected in our human spirituality.' In an epilogue to the book he remarks:

> Although perhaps recently underestimated, the psychodynamic and social aspects of mental illness have held a respected place in the history of American psychiatry. Its spiritual aspects, however, have not. Psychiatry has not only neglected but actively ignored the issue of spirituality.

He then alludes to the confusion between 'spirituality' and 'religion' and consequent misinterpretation which has contributed to this neglect.

SPIRITUAL CARE: NURSING

Over the last few years much work has been done in hospitals on care planning. This has more recently been introduced as standard practice in residential and nursing homes. Recent work has been directed towards developing care plans which will ensure that good quality care is delivered in such settings. Good quality care takes into account the physical, emotional and spiritual dimensions of health. Most care-givers are familiar with recognising, implementing and evaluating physical and emotional care; the spiritual aspect is more difficult to identify and assess. Mary Nathan, speaking at a meeting of the Spirituality Interest Group of the Royal College of Psychiatrists, described work she has done at the West London Mental Health Trust studying the perceptions of spiritual care in patients and the nurses who care for them. She also looked at whether or not mental health nurses feel sufficiently competent to assess and provide spiritual care to their clients. She has also looked at the possible barriers to provision of spiritual care.

Her findings showed that nurses had a lack of clarity with the concept of spirituality, which was most often thought of as related to meeting patients' religious needs. They identified a lack of training in this area and were unclear as to who should be responsible for this aspect of care.

Patients, in contrast, related spiritual care more to qualities of life and recovery. Nurses demonstrated a lack of confidence and expertise regarding spiritual care, but did express an interest in undertaking training when provided. Two of the main barriers identified were the lack of clarity of the concept and the confusion of religion and spirituality. Education was seen as an important means of overcoming barriers and using positive attitudes towards self and others in implementing care interventions that address the whole person.

Care in many contexts, such as hospital, residential and nursing homes, and even at home with homecare, has become so task-orientated that there seems to be no time left for relatedness. How often in the past has a particular home help or care assistant become a real friend to the person with dementia? Real mourning follows the death or the removal of a particular carer. With the time-conscious, task-orientated carer will this ever be the same? One hopes so or our own lives in later dependency will be bleak indeed.

CARE PLAN GUIDANCE

In 2000 the CCOA Dementia Group and Faith in Elderly People drew together much work on meeting the spiritual needs of those with dementia into a set of guidelines for care staff.[21] Two project workers, Gaynor Hammond and Laraine Moffitt, from Leeds and Newcastle respectively, wrote this to 'help staff understand the nature of spiritual needs and how to meet them, and arises out of work with care of older people, especially people with dementia'. The booklet aims to cultivate an approach which weaves spiritual care throughout the whole of care-giving. In this way it exemplifies Tom Kitwood's concept of person-centred care for the whole person in the entirety of their care needs. As they point out in the conclusion of the booklet: 'By acknowledging the spiritual dimension within all care practice, it may be easier for staff to justify why bathing a certain resident took longer today than usual – it may be that today the bathing met a need at the deepest level.' This work has been further developed into a holistic *Training Manual for Care Homes* by Gaynor Hammond.[22] We accept unquestioningly that bathing a young child may be a time of very important interpersonal communication. Why is it assumed that this possibility disappears as we become adults? Many have written about the deep spiritual understanding and responsiveness in those with severe learning disabilities. Why do we assume that the onset of dementia immediately destroys this essential part of human existence? Much that has been written about person-centred care for those with dementia applies to everyone in a care-receiving situation. Those with dementia are the least able to express their needs and thus have become a focus for attention. It is sad that in early part of the 21st century there are still many being 'cared for' in situations where their spiritual needs are ignored or not even acknowledged.

RELIGIOUS PRACTICE

The Prince of Wales[23] has pointed to the irony of asking a patient on admission to hospital to which religion they belong and then ignoring all that their religion may bring them in terms of how they understand and cope with illness. Religious observance may be one way to meet a spiritual need, but there may be others, even for a person of faith. Severe dementia, however, does not prevent a person responding appropriately and with great benefit to religious observance. Rituals and symbols are important, but those visiting in this capacity must be prepared to be flexible and expect the unexpected. Eileen Shamy[7] comments:

> Sometimes people hearing of our communion services will contest the whole thing on the grounds that the residents will not know what they are doing. Those who have witnessed and participated in these services would refute that. Very wonderful things happen. One day a most refined and well-spoken woman received the bread and wine very reverently and then burst out enthusiastically, 'Boy, that was good!'

As pointed out by Malcolm Goldsmith,[9] in 1981 Brown and Ellor stated the view that feelings remain intact and appropriate in people with Alzheimer's disease.[24] For those with a faith in a personal relationship with their God, surely it is arrogant to assume that they have been forgotten as well as forgetting so much themselves. Many people feel forgotten by their own faith communities (*see* Case Study 14.4).

Case Study 14.4

A Jewish patient was supported by the psychiatric team for the elderly. He had been an elder in the synagogue and the life of their religious community had been very important to him and his wife. They were distressed and lonely because none of the congregation of the synagogue ever visited them once he was unable to attend the synagogue himself because of his dementia.

PERSON-CENTRED CARE AND SPIRITUAL NEEDS

People have different personalities, needs, interests, preferences and, above all, different feelings about themselves and the world around them. Different types of dementing illnesses react with different personalities to produce unique situations. No one solution or set of rules will be right for everyone. Person-centred care focuses on the individual. Iain McGregor and Janet Bell[25] challenged the widely held beliefs that people with dementia cannot make choices, that they wander aimlessly and lose their ability for new learning. They point out that a well-designed environment can minimise dangers and thus allow residents to make decisions for themselves about how they spend their day. They acknowledge that this may be impossibly exhausting for a carer on their own, but in a specialist unit the result is a dynamic community with much interaction and group control.

Aimless wandering can be another misperceived expectation of those caring for people with advanced dementia. I once heard a very moving story about wandering that was misinterpreted with near-disastrous results (*see* Case Study 14.5). Another patient of my own was apparently aggressive with an elderly, lady but again his actions were misinterpreted (*see* Case Study 14.6).

Case Study 14.5

A man lived in a residential home. The night staff noticed that he wandered at night. Concern was becoming greater when observation revealed that he always went to a particular female resident's room. Discussion followed about the need for sedation or more draconian measures at this 'sexual' behaviour disorder. Fortunately, it was suggested that he was observed in detail first. On several nights he was observed to enter the old lady's room and bend down near to the head of her bed. He looked at her clock, read the time and then returned to his own room. A clock with a clear dial at his own bedside precluded the need for any more drastic measures.

Case Study 14.6

A man with advanced dementia was nursed in a special hospital unit for those with challenging behaviour. At the time of the Gulf War when much gunfire and bombing featured on the national news, he started trying to escape from the unit, dragging a female patient with him. With patience it was established that he was convinced the building was under fire and he was trying to escape, rescuing the lady with him.

An appreciation of the individual and his or her life experience and identity can help in all aspects of care, particularly those with dementia.

CONCLUSIONS

Returning to my introduction, although spirituality can be defined in many ways. I like the following:

> Spirituality can be described as a search for that which gives meaning and identity to a person's life and the wider world. Dementia does not destroy the ability to experience and appreciate the world about the person.[21]

This is well illustrated by Paul Wilson, writing in *Spirituality and Ageing*,[26] and relates to several of the points made in this chapter (*see* Case Study 14.7).

Case Study 14.7

The door opened and I was greeted by Alan and Barbara. Alan took me through the kitchen and stopped at his wife's activity table. On it were simple jigsaws, crayons, paper and materials. Alan told me how Barbara (the names are pseudonyms) spent an hour or so at a time at the table. He celebrated all she could do. As we spoke a video of Pavarotti was playing in the lounge. We stood and watched as Barbara joyfully danced, totally unaware of or inhibited by our presence. Alan spoke of her love of music and the enjoyment she received from the video, dancing and singing along to it. He expressed the hope that one day she would play the piano again. We sat down in the lounge and Barbara, the homemaker, went around all the pictures in the room, telling me about each one in great detail, but unfortunately, her speech was jumbled. Barbara has dementia.

I feel I can do no better than sum up the message of this chapter in Paul Wilson's words:

> Care-giving is thus more than the provision of a safe environment and communication with others; it is also the provision of spiritual care to nurture the person in the journey within and pastoral care to nurture the person in the journey above.

He quotes Buckland,[27] who talks of the 'fragile web of well-being' which is made up of strands of strength and positive experience. A living environment needs to take into account the effects that change and the ageing process are having on the person. Their values are developed in the core of their being by interacting with their experience and environment over the whole of their life. These values must be built into care-giving so that the person does not find him- or herself in an environment foreign to their lifestyle. We must remember that the person, however hidden from us by the fog of dementia, is still there and can still appreciate their surroundings. As Alison Froggatt so tellingly puts it in her book with Eileen Shamy:[6]

> The sacrament of the present moment has particular poignancy in dementia, for most happenings may be forgotten soon afterwards. But the rose smells just as sweet NOW, and the birds on the bird table are squabbling NOW and we can laugh.

Above all, we should learn to love those we care for. As Peter Huxham[28] points out, relationships are the only things which change people. We accept that principle in the care of children, but it applies throughout life. As the children's story quoted by Huxham so tellingly illustrates, loving relationships are essential to well-being.

> 'What is real' asked the Rabbit one day, when they were lying side by side near the nursery fender, because Nana came to tidy the room. 'Does it mean having things that buzz inside you and a stick-out handle?'

> 'Real isn't how you are made' said the Skin Horse. 'It's a thing that happens to you. When a child loves you for a long, long time, not just to play with but REALLY loves you, then you become real.'

> (From *The Velveteen Rabbit* by Margery Williams[29])

Spiritual aspects of dementia include the meeting of spiritual needs, but it is also essential to recognise the need in all humans for a 'sacred space' and the help needed to preserve or recreate such a space. A friend recently talked about her adjustment to retirement, including the adjustment to less 'doing' and more time for 'being'. Laraine Moffitt[30] compares religion as the 'doing' and spirituality as the 'being'. She suggests that learning to attend to someone's spiritual needs requires a shift of emphasis from helping them to *do* something, to providing the environment to allow them to *be*.

Key points

➤ Spirituality is the search for the meaning of life; religion is one way of conducting the search.

➤ Spiritual needs can be attended to by truly individualised care.

➤ Persons with dementia are indeed persons with emotions and feelings.

➤ Person-centred care is essential for well-being, especially in dementia care.

➤ Much current practice and legislation on dementia care does not take account of the spiritual dimension or person-centred care.

➤ Advanced dementia does not preclude enjoyment, loving relationships or creativity.

➤ People who are members of a faith community need to have continuing contact and will benefit from participation in faith practice.

REFERENCES

1 Swinton J. *Spirituality and Mental Health Care*. London and Philadelphia: Jessica Kingsley Publishers; 2001.
2 Krishna Mohan K. Spirituality and well-being: an overview. In: Cornelissen M (ed). *Consciousness and its Transformation*. Pondicherry: Sri Aurobindo Ashram Press; 2001.
3 Stoter D. *Spiritual Aspects of Health Care*. London: Mosby; 1995.
4 Kitwood T. *Dementia Reconsidered*. Buckingham: Open University Press; 1997.
5 Froggatt A. Self-awareness in early dementia. In: Gearing B, Johnson M, Heller T (eds). *Mental Health Problems in Old Age*. Buckingham: Open University Press; 1988.
6 Froggatt A, Shamy E. *Dementia: a Christian perspective*. Derby: CCOA Publications; 1998.
7 Shamy E. *More than Body, Brain and Breath*. New Zealand: ColCom Press; 1997. (Edited version by Albert Jewell under title *A Guide to the Spiritual Dimension of Care for people with Alzheimer's Disease and Related Dementia*. London and Bristol, PA: Jessica Kingsley Publishers; 2003.)
8 Kitwood T. Cultures of care: tradition and change. In: Kitwood T, Benson S (eds). *The New Culture of Dementia Care*. London: Hawker Publications; 1995.
9 Goldsmith M. *Hearing the Voice of People with Dementia*. London and Bristol, PA: Jessica Kingsley Publishers; 1996.
10 Killick J (ed). *You are Words*. London: Hawker Publications; 1997.

11 Killick J, Cordonnier C (eds). *Openings*. London: Hawker Publications; 2000.

12 Bryden C. *Dancing with Dementia*. London: Jessica Kingsley Publishers; 2005.

13 Taylor R. *Alzheimer's from the Inside Out*. Baltimore, MD: Health Professions Press; 2007.

14 Department of Health. *Care Homes for Older People: national minimum standards*. 3rd ed. London: DoH; 2003.

15 Caritas Social Action Network. *'Its still ME, Lord ...', a film exploring spirituality and dementia* [DVD]. London: CSAN; 2009.

16 Johnson AM, Hickman Morris H. *Understanding the Needs of Older People*. Leveson Centre Paper 1, 2000.

17 Office for National Statistics. *Living in Britain: results from the general household survey 1994*. Newport: ONS; 1996.

18 Crossley D. Religious experience within mental illness. *British Journal of Psychiatry*. 1995; **166**: 284–6.

19 Sims ACP. 'Psyche' – spirit as well as mind? *British Journal of Psychiatry*. 1994; **165**: 441–6.

20 Peck SM. *Further Along the Road Less Travelled*. London: Simon & Schuster; 1993.

21 Hammond G, Moffitt L. *Guidelines for Care Plans*. Leeds: CCOA Publications and Faith in Elderly People; 2002. Preface and p. 2.

22 Hammond G. *Training Manual for Care Homes*. Leeds: Faith in Elderly People; 2009.

23 HRH The Prince of Wales. 150th Anniversary Lecture. *British Journal of Psychiatry*. 1991; **159**: 763–8.

24 Brown M, Ellor J. An approach to the treatment of symptoms caused by cognitive disorders in the aged. *Salud Publications*: **23**. Cincinatti, OH; 1981.

25 McGregor I, Bell J. Buzzing with life, energy and drive. *Journal of Dementia Care*. 1994; **1**(6): 20–1.

26 Wilson P. Memory, personhood and faith. In: Jewell A (ed). *Spirituality and Ageing*. London: Jessica Kingsley Publishers; 1999.

27 Buckland S. Well-being personality and residential care. In: Kitwood T, Benson S (eds). *The New Culture of Dementia Care*. London: Hawker Publications; 1995.

28 Huxham P. I'm not very religious, but ... In: Corley G (ed). *Older People and their Needs*. London: Whurr Publishers; 2000.

29 Williams M. *The Velveteen Rabbit*. London: Heinemann; 1922.

30 Moffitt L. Helping to re-create a personal sacred space. *Journal of Dementia Care*. 1996; **4**(3): 19–21.

FURTHER READING

➤ Brooker D. *Person-centred Dementia Care*. London and Philadelphia: Jessica Kingsley Publishers; 2007.

➤ Allen, Reverend B (ed). *Religious Practice and People with Dementia: a resource for carers*. Derby: CCOA Publications; 2002. (See www.ccoa.org.uk for this and other related titles.)

➤ Downs M, Bowers B (eds). *Excellence in Dementia Care, Research into Practice*. Buckingham: Open University Press; 2008.

➤ Kitwood T, Buckland S, Petre T. *Brighter Futures*. Oxford: Anchor Housing Association; 1995.

➤ Orchard H (ed), *Spirituality in Health Care Contexts*. London and Philadelphia: Jessica Kingsley Publishers; 2001.

➤ Post SG. *The Moral Challenge of Alzheimer Disease*. Baltimore, MD: Johns Hopkins University Press; 1995.

CHAPTER 15

Comprehensive and integrated mental health services for people with dementia

Ben Boyd and Sue Barton

INTRODUCTION

Previous chapters will have reported on the growing elderly population and the burgeoning expectations that have accompanied a remarkable period of development in the UK over the last 30 years. They will also have touched upon how mental health services have changed in that time, with increasing focus on care in the community and subsequent de-institutionalisation. Notwithstanding the recent economic downturn, these factors have resulted in one further trend, increasing pressure on public finances to deliver specialist mental health services for older people (MHSOP).

This is set in a strategic environment where funding for mental health services still relies on an outdated payments mechanism and a shift from inspection to regulation with the advent of the Care Quality Commission.

At present there is no definitive blueprint for how MHSOP should be constructed and delivered. In contrast, and often in direct competition, with mental health services for working-age adults, a plethora of central government targets have resulted in significant investment and a uniformity of service elements across the country. Arguably, this has been a double-edged sword for MHSOP. On the one hand, it allowed freedom to develop services where local knowledge of the community was the driver for development. On the other, it has offered little incentive and much risk for commissioners to invest in services where there is an absence of national consensus.

This chapter will consider the historical context and main policy drivers that have influenced MHSOP, looking at how they have evolved and the impact of this on service development and delivery now. It will also consider the impact of the separation of people by age within a mental health service.

HISTORICAL CONTEXT

In the first half of the 20th century psychiatric care for all people in Britain was provided in large hospitals known as county asylums. Within these institutions older people with mental disorders were typically thought of as senile, given no hope of recovery and were housed in the now infamous 'back wards' where psychiatrists rarely ventured.[1]

In the 1950s studies began to emerge offering a new perspective on the older population, not only differentiating between dementia and other mental health problems, but finding that the majority of older people with some conditions recovered enough to be discharged from the asylum.[2] In the US a seminal study by the National Institute of Mental Health[3] concluded that senility was due to specific disorders and not simply a consequence of ageing. And by the end of the decade, the World Health Organization had recognised the specific mental health needs of older people.[4]

It was also becoming evident that life expectancy in the UK was increasing, with more older people requiring hospital care within the maturing NHS. Subsequently a new branch of medicine evolved specialising in the physical conditions that often accompanied ageing: geriatrics. By the 1970s some of these geriatricians were organising psycho-geriatric units due to the large number of older people in their care with mental health problems and who their psychiatrist colleagues were apparently not interested in looking after.[5] This lack of interest may have been common, but it was by no means universal: some psychiatrists were organising their own services locally for older people,[6,7] and co-operating closely with geriatricians. By 1978 The Royal College of Psychiatrists had formed a section for Psychiatry of Old Age, though this was not officially recognised by the Department of Health for another decade.[8]

Government policy of the day reflected this evolution of services, and perhaps the tensions between and within agencies, recommending what it saw as sufficient psychiatric hospital resources for older people and trying to delineate the responsibilities of geriatricians, psychiatrists and social services for people with dementia.[9] Government, it would seem, was forced into the role of referee rather than that of moderniser. That said, the results must have pleased those in power; less than a decade later government policy was fully behind the development of specialist psychiatric services for older people.[10]

MHSOP in the 1990s had not only become commonplace but had moved beyond specialist medical staff and out of the hospital. Community mental health teams (CMHTs), comprised mainly of nurses but including some other disciplines such as occupational therapists, had been developed in many localities,[11] but often operated very differently. Helpfully, a joint initiative between geriatricians and psychiatrists produced guidance for the operation and resourcing of MHSOP.[12] Within the guidance it recommended close working arrangements between geriatricians and old age psychiatrists. And for each population of 20 000 people over 65 years of age it placed an old age psychiatrist at the centre of a discrete service, supported by a CMHT and day hospital places and hospital beds for both people with dementia and older people with other mental health difficulties. Updated in 1992, this guidance underpinned the recruitment of old age psychiatrists,[13] and therefore gave incentive, as well as direction, for service development (Table 15.1).

Table 15.1 Recommended resources for people over 65

Medical resources	Community and other staffing	Hospital-based resources
1.0 wte consultant per 10 000	1.0 wte nurse per 5000	10 acute psychiatric beds per 10 000, preferably on district general hospital site
Emphasis on home visits	1.0 wte occupational therapist per 10 000	
Included in junior, senior registrar and clinical assistants training posts	1.0 wte physiotherapist per 20 000	25–30 long stay beds (including respite) per 10 000
0.5 to 1.0 wte secretary per 10 000	1.0 wte clinical psychologist per 20 000	2–3 day hospital places per 1000
	Access to speech and language therapy	

wte = whole time equivalent
Royal College of Psychiatrists (RCPsych) Guidelines for regional advisers on consultant posts in the psychiatry of old age, 1992[13]

The impact of this should not be underestimated: it set the boundaries for older peoples services at age 65, not only the retirement age for men in the UK but the age when the incidence of dementia within the population rises sharply. And not to be overlooked, in 1980 the number of old age psychiatrists in the UK was around 120,[14] but by the year 2000 their number had grown to over 540,[15] with presumably something like the attendant services recommended above.

POLICY CONTEXT

Shortly after its election in 1997, the Labour Government embarked on its promised reforms of the NHS, with the overarching aim to improve the health of the nation and reduce the inequalities in society that contributed to poor health. The mechanisms to achieve this would be National Service Frameworks (NSFs). The NSFs were essentially standards for services that people should expect to receive in any part of England; other parts of the UK had devolved responsibility for healthcare and produced their own guidance. The NSFs were aimed at the 'big' healthcare issues, namely cancer, heart disease, mental health problems and diabetes, or where it was thought elements of society had significant health issues, such as older people and children. They not only offered guidance on how services could be configured, based on best evidence agreed by an external reference group, but set government targets, for example, a reduction of 20% in suicide by 2010. The NSFs were accompanied in 2000 by *the NHS Plan*, a document that promised to change the NHS from a 1940s healthcare system to one that was fit for the 21st century. It outlined the government's intention to increase funding hugely and over the following decade deliver 7000 extra hospital beds, new intermediate care services, over 100 new hospitals, 7500 more consultants, 2000 more GPs and 20 000 extra nurses.

Significantly, the first of the NSFs to be launched was for mental health in 1999; however, on page 3 of the document it clearly excluded MHSOP.

> This National Service Framework focuses on the *mental health needs of working age adults* up to 65.
>
> (National Service Framework for Mental Health, 1999)

Arguably this made sense from a policy perspective, reflecting the separate services that had developed over the previous two decades. MHSOP had received additional investment during this time and from the authors' experience working age adult (WAA) services had felt somewhat depleted as a result; the majority of staff recruited to MHSOP had worked in WAA or in teams who catered for both populations.

The NSF Mental Health resulted in significant additional funding for WAA services (*see* Table 15.2). Allowing for inflation, the national spend on adult

Table 15.2 Government investment in WAA Mental Health Services in England

Year	Real-term investment in £ billions				Percentage increase
	Reported investment	Estimated unreported investment	Total investment	Annual increase	
2001/02	3.769	0.151	3.920		
2002/03	4.072	0.257	4.329	0.409	10.4%
2003/04	4.437	0.037	4.474	0.146	3.4%
2004/05	4.942	0.051	4.993	0.519	11.6%
2005/06	5.065	0.244	5.308	0.315	6.3%
2006/07	5.258	0.181	5.439	0.131	2.5%
2007/08	5.650	0.018	5.668	0.228	4.2%
2008/09	5.849	0.043	5.892	0.224	4.0%
Increase 2001/02 to 2008/09		1.972		1.972	50.3%

2008/2009 National Survey of Investment in Adult Mental Health Services

mental health services in England rose by £1.972 billion from £3.920 billion in 2001/02 to £5.892 billion in 2008/09.[16]

The NSF Mental Health was followed by complementary guidance[17] that set out service specifications for meeting some of its key objectives, namely improving access to services and providing more significant community support, including 24-hour crisis teams. In much the same way as the joint initiative between geriatricians and old age psychiatrists over a decade earlier had, this document laid out detailed information on how many staff for a designated adult population would be required to provide the new services and how they should operate. However, there are some interesting differences between the two. The 2001 guidance referenced a great deal more published evidence about the services it described, including outcomes. The emphasis for investment was not on psychiatrists but on other mental health disciplines. It was a government-owned document written with the intention of advising local commissioners how to invest the funding that was now starting to flow from the NHS Plan. Though its language was a little softer than the NSF for Mental Health with respect to older people, it was still clearly aimed at services for the under-65 population.

All of this investment and national initiative was in stark contrast to the guidance produced for MHSOP. In 2001 the government launched the NSF for Older People,[18] aimed at improving health and social care for all older people. Though many of the statistics within the document used age 65 and over to define older people, it was made clear that chronological age alone did not determine the target population and suggested the older person could be anything from 50 upwards, depending on their circumstances. It gave eight standards, including one for mental health, as outlined below (*see* Box 15.1), and with these set milestones for local commissioners and providers to have achieved specific objectives.

From this brief overview it can be seen that, as with the NSF Mental Health, the government was directing commissioners to establish new specialist services, in this case for intermediate care, stroke and falls, where they did not already exist.

If one of the aims of the NSF for older people was to seek to address inconsistencies in care provided to older people with mental health difficulties, then it seems that this has not been achieved. A postal survey of old age psychiatrists undertaken three years after publication by Tucker *et al.*[19] in 2007 concluded that there were considerable differences in community teams, with less than a quarter of the psychiatrists considering that community provision was adequate.

The Mental Health standard in the NSF for older people focused on older people with depression and dementia as these were the largest sub-groups within the older population. For people with psychosis interestingly it indicated:

Box 15.1   Eight standards for improving health and social care for older people in England

Standard 1: Rooting out age discrimination	NHS services will be provided, regardless of age, on the basis of clinical need alone. Social care services will not use age in their eligibility criteria or policies, to restrict access to available services.
Standard 2: Person-centred care	NHS and social care services treat older people as individuals and enable them to make choices about their own care. This is achieved through the single assessment process, integrated commissioning arrangements and integrated provision of services, including community equipment and continence services.
Standard 3: Intermediate care	Older people will have access to a new range of services at home or in designated care settings, to promote their independence by providing enhanced services from the NHS and councils to prevent unnecessary hospital admission and effective rehabilitation services to enable early discharge from hospital and to prevent premature or unnecessary admission to long-term residential care.
Standard 4: General hospital care	Older people's care in hospital is delivered through appropriate specialist care and by hospital staff who have the right set of skills to meet their needs.
Standard 5: Stroke	The NHS will take action to prevent strokes, working in partnership with other agencies. People who are thought to have had a stroke will have access to diagnostic services, be treated by a specialist stroke service and with their carers, participate in a multidisciplinary programme of secondary prevention and rehabilitation.
Standard 6: Falls	The NHS, in partnership with councils, takes action to prevent falls and reduce resultant fractures or other injuries in their populations of older people. Older people who have fallen receive effective treatment and rehabilitation and, with their carers, receive advice on prevention, through a specialised falls service.

| Standard 7: Mental health in older people | Older people who have mental health problems have access to integrated mental health services, provided by the NHS and councils to ensure effective diagnosis, treatment and support, for them and for their carers. |
| Standard 8: The promotion of health and active life in older age | The health and well-being of older people is promoted through a coordinated programme of action led by the NHS with support from councils. |

NSF for Older People 2001[18]

Where an older person has severe mental illness due to a psychotic illness such as schizophrenia, they will require the packages of care set out in the NSF for Mental Health and the same standards should apply as for working age adults. For these people care should be provided within the framework of the Care Programme Approach.

(NSF for Older People 2001[18])

This would infer that at least some older people should have access to the new services being rapidly established in WAA services. However, it fails to clarify whether these services should be duplicated or that older people should have access to WAA services. If either was intended then no one, it seems, communicated this effectively and the upper age limit of 65 remained firmly in place. It can only be assumed, but it seems likely that the government somehow did communicate that there would be no new funding for MHSOP.

Indeed, the milestones set for MHSOP were relatively speaking investment free, directed as they were towards establishing agreed multi-agency protocols for the management of dementia and depression, and integrated working across health and social care. This is not to say that this document prevented commissioners funding MHSOP, but in neither NSF Mental Health nor NSF Older People was there any incentive to direct additional funding toward this specialty. Attempts have been made to rectify this situation, indicating that if nothing else the government at least recognised the problem. Two major guidance documents were released (*Securing Better Mental Health Services for Older People 2005*,[20] *Everybody's Business 2005* [21]). Whilst they were influential, neither was able to address the difficult issue of establishing a national consensus on service configuration or performance information to give incentive for commissioners to release extra funding for MHSOP.[22,23] The additional guidance stressed the need to provide services as close to the service user as possible, with the focus being on the service going to the service user.

The one area where performance indicators were established as a result of NSF Older People was in relation to integrated working within older people's CMHTs. The drive for this pre-dated the NSFs and arose as a result of two separate national inspections of services in England. The inspectors found that where teams worked collaboratively across health and social care boundaries older people received better care packages.[24,25] The subsequent performance indicators are outlined in Box 15.2.

This would result in CMHTs finding one way of working that tied together several disparate national strategies: Care Management within Social care, Care Programme Approach for mental health and the Single Assessment Process for Older People, not to mention the issue of NHS teams and council social services departments often having different paperwork or electronic record systems. Unsurprisingly, the success of this has been doubtful. Despite all areas in England reporting that they have achieved these six indicators, the Healthcare Commission found that on closer inspection the actual success rate could be nearer 40%.[23]

Box 15.2 CMHT integration criteria

➤ The community mental health team has at least two different disciplines from health and a social care worker who is suitably experienced to carry out initial assessment on behalf of the team, meeting at least weekly (face to face or by other electronic means).

➤ Referrals to all members of the community mental health team can be made through a single point of access.

➤ Individuals within this team produce and share a current summary record

➤ Individuals within this team use a common assessment process

➤ Individuals within this team carry out a common care planning methodology

➤ Individuals within this team carry out integrated care coordination**

** Integrated care coordination means that no additional assessment is required for accessing health or social care resources beyond the usual resource gatekeeping processes. The care coordinator, whether employed by health or social care agencies, should be able to access all mental healthcare and social care services without the service user having to undergo any further assessment for eligibility. (CMHT Integration (Older People), Healthcare Commission, 2007)

In spite of the confusion surrounding national strategy, MHSOP across England had been setting up new community services. And, interestingly, there is a commonality to these developments if not the uniformity that can be ascribed to WAA services. Across the country MHSOP have been setting up memory assessment clinics and teams that support older people in care homes, general hospitals and out-of-office hours,[27] although in the authors' experience these have often been funded through depleting more traditional, hospital-based resources such as day hospitals and in-patient beds.[28] The NSF Older People had been clear about one thing, services it recommended should be 'community oriented'.

It would be natural to think pessimistically about the future of MHSOP given the recent history. However, new national initiatives give some degree of optimism, even if the economic recession the UK has been experiencing since 2007 does not. The government released the National Dementia Strategy (NDS) in February 2009.[29] This strategy proposes a whole system strategy for people with a diagnosis of dementia and acknowledges the challenges that the increased demographics of an ageing population poses. It sets out a five-year programme to transform dementia services across England, identifying 17 key objectives in addition to an implementation plan. The strategy was launched with an additional £150 million of funding for primary care trusts, but as this funding was not 'ring-fenced' and simply included in an uplift of finances to meet inflationary pressures, it is difficult to know what direct impact it will have on services.

The strategy defines three main areas which care agencies should focus on:
1 improving awareness of dementia
2 early diagnosis and support to people with dementia and their carers
3 higher quality care for everybody with a diagnosis of dementia.

(National Dementia Strategy 2009[29])

This strategy is to be welcomed as it clearly identifies the changes required across the whole system of health, social care and the voluntary sector if we are to more fully meet the complex needs of people with dementia and their carers. It has also been designed to establish evidence toward effective service configuration and produce performance information against which commissioners can be measured. These two latter elements will be vital in securing the necessary funding to turn the ambitions of this strategy into tangible improvements in care services.

WHAT ARE THE KEY COMPONENTS OF A COMPREHENSIVE AND INTEGRATED MENTAL HEALTH SERVICE FOR PEOPLE WITH DEMENTIA?

The key components of a comprehensive and integrated service for people with dementia are many and varied but given the range of agencies involved a focal point for commissioning, involvement and service provision is vital. They can

Box 15.3   Components of an integrated dementia service

Improving awareness	➤ A local health promotion strategy that engages the wider community in assisting people with dementia to navigate day-to-day life and encourages help-seeking behaviour for those worried about having dementia. ➤ A single point of contact for good quality information and advice that is non-threatening and easily accessed. ➤ Involving people with dementia and their carers in community development and the design of care services.
Early diagnosis and support	➤ A better than novice level understanding of dementia for all mainstream health and social care workers. Intermediate or higher level understanding of dementia for all mainstream health and social care workers directly involved in the assessment of people likely to have dementia. ➤ An early intervention approach to dementia in the local health and social care community aimed at reducing the duration of undetected dementia. ➤ Clear, well-publicised protocols for referral to specialist diagnostic services through an easy to access single point of entry. ➤ Specialist diagnostic services where all staff have expert level understanding of dementia. ➤ Specialist diagnostic services that are adequately resourced to meet the demands within the population and provide 'one-stop-shop' access to health and social care resources. ➤ Ongoing support for people where a diagnosis is uncertain but they remain concerned about their memory. ➤ Criteria for accessing health and social care services that ensures early access to support and not simply rationed on the basis of those with highest level of existing disability. ➤ Care co-ordination by a member of staff with expert level of understanding from the point of diagnosis through to a point where this ends by mutual consent.
Higher quality care	➤ Access to services that retain the individual's sense of value as a person through employment, leisure, occupation, the arts, life history and advocacy. ➤ Services that engage with carers and families and not simply attempt to replace them. ➤ Services that are regularly measured for quality of experience and care standards, e.g. through Dementia Care Mapping ➤ Access to 24-hour, 7 days a week intensive community services designed to prevent crisis and maintain the person at home. ➤ Access to a range of high quality residential services including acute mental health care. ➤ Better than novice up to expert level understanding of dementia range of certified training for all staff in direct care settings where people with dementia are cared for. ➤ Better than novice up to expert level of training for all staff in end of life care in residential settings and specialist services.

be grouped under headings suggested by the three main aims of the NDS, as shown in Box 15.3.

STRATEGIC CONTEXT

Prior to 2003, secondary health services in England, such as district hospital trusts, were commissioned by what is commonly known as a 'block' contract. A provider would receive a lump sum of money from the commissioning body, typically a primary care trust, based on the amount of services it offered. The key factors in determining how much the block contract was worth were the previous year's funding, adjustments for inflation, current cost pressures and any potential for cost improvement.

Payment by Results (PbR) aims to improve NHS finances by setting a fixed price, or tariff, for each individual case.[30] Tariffs are based on data comparisons from across the NHS on groups of similar treatment episodes. The data is then translated into 'currencies' that describe the treatment and, by comparing services across the country, costs can be extrapolated. This system has been implemented within general healthcare and has lead to a more accurate and fairer basis for funding.[22] It is set for implementation within mental health services in shadow form by 2011 and fully by 2013.

PbR would also support other major NHS reforms, foundation trusts (FTs) and Patient Choice;[31] the new funding arrangements offered an incentive, whereby FTs could recoup funds for spending elsewhere if they offered treatment at a cost below fixed tariffs or generate a surplus. With respect to patient choice, the funding would now follow the patient and equally allow the patient to choose a hospital where, for example, waiting lists were short. More recently, World Class Commissioning guidance has been produced[32] where a local joint strategic needs assessment is completed by commissioners. From this, plans are developed to improve investment that leads to greater gains in health and reduced inequality at best value rates for funding.

The environment is also affected by the changes in regulatory systems with the development of the Care Quality Commission (CQC). All NHS, social care and independent providers of care were required to register with the CQC by 2010 in order to operate legally in England. Rather than ensure high standards by inspection of services offered, the CQC will now expect care providers to produce evidence of quality based on patient experience and outcomes.[23]

Common strategic themes are emerging within the NHS, themes that MHSOP will have to embrace to ensure their survival and further development. Good quality information systems will be a prerequisite, not only to gather data on performance but also to ensure both patients and commissioners understand what services have to offer. Service delivery will have to become outcome focused and be able to articulate how these outcomes are being achieved without staff spending more time on bureaucracy than they do on direct patient care. Within mental health services information systems have traditionally been poor,[33] and within MHSOP this is compounded by a reticence toward a target-driven outcomes focused performance culture.

CONCLUSIONS

The changing environment of the NHS means that services to people with dementia have to adapt and change in order to maximise the benefits for the people that they serve – both service users and their carers. The National Dementia Strategy[29] provides an ideal opportunity to further develop services for this growing population. The strategy focuses on the need for the whole system of health, social care and the third sector to work together, along with the community they serve in order to develop an environment for people with dementia to live as full a life as possible.

It is essential that in this changing environment we learn lessons from the past and build services that focus on the individual and their specific needs.

The current financial climate means that we have to undertake this continued improvement in an environment where resources are tight. This provides an interesting challenge, particularly because of the increased demand, but also provides an additional incentive for us to develop innovative solutions to meet the needs of people with dementia and their families.

One of the major challenges that remains is to address the understanding of people within society about the nature of dementia so that some of the improvements in the quality of life of people who have been given a diagnosis of dementia come from how we all react and respond to them as well as how services are continued to be improved to meet their needs.

Key points

➤ Leadership for the development of old age mental health services initially came from physicians and psychiatrists.

➤ More recently national guidance in the National Service Frameworks has been ambiguous about the needs of older people with functional mental health problems.

➤ There is now, however, a National Dementia Strategy.

➤ Developments for Mental Health Services for Older People have rarely been associated with earmarked resources.

➤ Development has therefore often demanded the creative redeployment of existing resources against a background of rapidly rising demand (and recently more severely constrained finances).

REFERENCES

1 Arie T, Isaacs AD. The development of psychiatric services for the elderly in Britain. In: Post F, Isaacs AD (eds). *Studies in Geriatric Psychiatry*. Chichester: John Wiley & Sons; 1977. pp. 241–6.

2 Roth M. The natural history of mental disorder in old age. *Journal of Mental Science*. 1955; **101**: 281–301.

3 Butler RN. Psychiatry and the elderly: an overview. *American Journal of Psychiatry*. 1975; **132**: 893–900.

4 World Health Organization. *Mental Health Problems of Ageing and the Aged: sixth report of the expert committee on Mental Health*. Technical report series 171. New York: WHO; 1959.

5 Godber C. Conflict and collaboration between geriatric medicine and psychiatry. In: Isaacs B (ed). *Recent Advances in Geriatric Medicine*. London: Churchill Livingstone; 1978. pp. 131–42.

6 Arie T. The first year of the Goodmayes psychiatric service for old people. *Lancet*. 1970; **ii**: 1179–82.

7 Pitt B. *Psychogeriatrics*. London: Churchill Livingstone; 1974.

8 Benbow S. Training requirements for old age psychiatrists in the UK. In: Copeland J, Abou-Saleh MT, Blazer D (eds). *Principles and Practice of Geriatric Psychiatry*. 2nd ed. Chichester: John Wiley & Sons; 2002. pp. 791–3.

9 Department of Health and Social Security. *Services for Mental Illness Related to Old Age*. DHSS Circular HM (72). London: HMSO; 1972.

10 Department of Health and Social Security. *Growing Older*. London: HMSO; 1981.

11 Dening T. Community psychiatry of old age: a UK perspective. *International Journal of Geriatric Psychiatry*. 1992; **7**: 757–66.

12 Royal College of Physicians and the Royal College of Psychiatrists. *Care of Elderly People with Mental Illness. Specialist services and medical training*. London: Royal College of Physicians, Royal College of Psychiatrists; 1989.

13 The Royal College of Psychiatrists. *Mental Health of the Nation – the contribution of psychiatry*. Council Report CR16. London: RCP; 1992. Editors' note: more up-to-date guidance is available on the Royal College of Psychiatrists website, www.rcpsych. ac.uk

14 Wattis J, Wattis L, Arie T. Psychogeriatrics: a national survey of a new branch of psychiatry. *British Medical Journal*. 1981; **282**: 1529–33.

15 Audini B, Lelliot P, Bannerjee S, *et al*. *Old Age Psychiatric Day Hospital Survey. Final Report*. London: The Royal College of Psychiatrists' Research Unit; 2001.

16 Department of Health. *2008/09 National Survey of Investment in Adult Mental Health Services*. London: DoH; 2009. Available at: www.dh.gov.uk/prod_consum_dh/ groups/dh_digitalassets/documents/digitalasset/dh_103198.pdf (accessed May 2011).

17 Department of Health. *The Mental Health Policy Implementation Guide*. London: DoH; 2001. Available at; www.dh.gov.uk/prod_consum_dh/groups/dh_digitalassets/@ dh/@en/documents/digitalasset/dh_4058960.pdf (accessed August 2011).

18 Department of Health. *National Service Framework for Older People*. London: DoH; 2001.

19 Tucker S, Baldwin R, Hughes J, *et al*. Old age mental health services in England: implementing the National Service Framework for Older People. *International Journal of Geriatric Psychiatry*. 2007; **22**: 211–17.

20 Department of Health. *Securing Better Mental Health Services for Older People*. London: DoH; 2005.

21 Department of Health (Care Services Improvement Partnership). *Everybody's Business. Integrated mental health service for older adults: a service development guide*. London: DoH; 2005.

22 Audit Commission. *The Right Result? Payment by results 2003–07*. London: Audit Commission; 2008. Available at: www.audit-commission.gov.uk/nationalstudies/healthcare/financialmanagement/Pages/therightresult.asp? (accessed May 2011).

23 Care Quality Commission. *A New System of Registration: guide for providers of healthcare or adult social care*. Newcastle upon Tyne: CQC; 2009. Available at: www.cqc.org.uk/_db/_documents/New_system_of_registration_Guide_for_providers_FINAL.pdf (accessed May 2011).

24 Healthcare Commission Indicators 2005 at: http://ratings.healthcarecommission.org.uk/Indicators_2005/Trust/Indicator/indicatorDescriptionShort.asp?indicatorId=3720 (accessed August 2011).

25 Healthcare Commission Indicators 2006 at: http://ratings2006.healthcarecommission.org.uk/Indicators_2006Nat/Trust/Indicator/indicatorDescriptionShort.asp?indicatorId=3232 (accessed August 2011).

26 Healthcare Commission Indicators 2007 at: http://ratings2007.healthcarecommission.org.uk/Indicators_2007Nat/Trust/Indicator/indicatorDescriptionShort.asp?indicatorId=3232 (accessed August 2011).

27 Healthcare Commission. *Equality in Later Life: A national study of older people's mental health services*. London: Healthcare Commission; 2009.

28 Boyd, B. Community mental health teams and specialist day services for older people: an integrated development. *Mental Health and Learning Disabilities Research*. 2006; 3: 21–37.

29 Department of Health. *Reforming NHS Financial Flows: introducing payment by results*. London: DoH; 2002. Available at: www.dh.gov.uk/en/Publicationsandstatistics/Publications/PublicationsPolicyAndGuidance/DH_4005300 (accessed May 2011).

30 Department of Health. *Delivering the NHS Plan: next steps on investment, next steps on reform*. London: DoH; 2002. Available at: www.dh.gov.uk/en/Publicationsandstatistics/Publications/PublicationsPolicyAndGuidance/DH_4005818 (accessed May 2011).

31 Department of Health. *World Class Commissioning: vision*. London: DoH; 2007. Available at: www.dh.gov.uk/en/Publicationsandstatistics/Publications/PublicationsPolicyAndGuidance/DH_080956 (accessed May 2011).

32 Dent E. A picture of progress. *Health Service Journal*. 2006; **116**(6021): 20–2.

33 Department of Health. *National Dementia Strategy*. London: DoH; 2009. Available at: www.dh.gov.uk/en/socialcare/deliveringadultsocialcare/olderpeople/nationaldementiastrategy/index.htm (accessed May 2011).

FURTHER READING

➤ Beecham J, Knapp M, Fernandez JL, *et al*. *Age Discrimination in Mental Health Services*. Personal Social Services Research Unit; 2008. Available at: www.pssru.ac.uk/pdf/dp2536.pdf (accessed May 2011).

➤ British Medical Association CCSC Psychiatry subcommittee. *Survey of BMA Members' Views on Mental Health Funding and Patient Care.* London: BMA; 2008. Available at: www.bma.org.uk/images/CCSCmentalhealthsurvey08_tcm41-173392.pdf (accessed May 2011).

➤ Centre for Policy on Ageing. *A Literature Review of the Likely Costs and Benefits of Legislation to Prohibit Age Discrimination in Health, Social Care and Mental Health Services and Definitions of Age Discrimination that might be Operationalised for Measurement.* London: CPA; 2007. Available at; www.cpa.org.uk/information/reviews/CPA-age_discrimination_costs_report.pdf (accessed May 2011).

CHAPTER 16

The role of service users and carers in helping to develop and improve services for people with dementia

Virginia Minogue

INTRODUCTION

Service user and carer engagement is an accepted element of much of health and social care activity and ranges from involvement in decisions about individual care to advocacy, research and education. Yet, people with dementia have been less engaged in the development and improvement of health and social care services. Involving people with dementia is often seen as a challenge because of the perceived difficulties in communication. However, it is worth noting that the majority of our communication with others is non-verbal, so speech, or lack of it, does not necessarily have to form a barrier. Carers of people with dementia have also been excluded from involvement in activity, though for different reasons, primarily time constraints, lack of recognition of carer's needs and perspectives on the carer's role. The fact that many people with dementia are also older people can add to the perception that there are constraints in engaging with them. Although Law *et al.*[1] found many examples of involvement and engagement with older people, they found that there were few examples of how engagement had changed services to reflect their wishes.

It is also important to note that of the 700 000 people with dementia in the UK[2] there are a significant, albeit small, number (approximately 18 000) of younger people amongst them. Their needs will be very different from those of the older population as their physical health may be better and levels of social inclusion higher.

WHY SHOULD PEOPLE WITH DEMENTIA BE INVOLVED IN DEVELOPING SERVICES?

Firstly, it is important to recognise that there are policy drivers which underpin public engagement in service development. However, there are also social and societal determinants which make it not only desirable but crucial that service users and carers are involved in the planning and delivery of current and future services. The increase in the population of older people that is anticipated in the next decade will increase the number of people with dementia who will require health and/or social care. It is, therefore, crucial that we understand more about their needs and wishes in order to provide timely and relevant services. People with dementia need to have the opportunity to express their views and be heard. They, and potentially their carers, are in the best position to identify their needs; services may then become more relevant and appropriate to meet those needs. Scientific knowledge about the condition has made early diagnosis of dementia more likely and this means that people with dementia want more information to enable them to understand what is happening to them and to plan accordingly. Carers have particular, and unique, expertise in the caring role. It is estimated that carers provide between 13.1 and 46.1 hours of informal care each week for older people with dementia, saving the UK economy £15 billion per year.[3]

Furthermore, it is known that age discrimination is a key concern in accessing health and social care, to the detriment of older people.[4] Lack of resources and funding, unmet need, poor quality services, cultural attitudes to older people and ageing are all issues leading to exclusion and discrimination. Although the national dementia strategy[2] has done much to address the shortfall in the quality of services for people with dementia, older people still face discrimination in other areas of their lives.

Policy context

There has been a raft of policy and guidance, emanating primarily from the Department of Health over the last 10 years, advocating patient and public involvement and engagement (PPI/PPE) in care and decisions about their treatment.[5-13] Yet, older adults often feel disenfranchised from making decisions about their own health and social care while professionals, and sometimes their own families, may believe they are not capable of a balanced judgement.[14] This can be born out of some of the symptoms of dementia-related illnesses such as memory loss, confusion, communication difficulties and loss of concentration. However, similar symptoms may be prevalent in other forms of mental illness but it is notable that the language used in discussing typologies of treatment and the intervention are different. It is routine to talk in terms of treatment based on a central concept of person-centred care, in working in general mental health services but the adoption of similar principles in treating people with dementia and older adults has been slower.[15,16]

Two early guidance documents espoused the view that the public should participate in decisions and policies that affect their health and shape health services.[5,6] *The NHS Plan*[7] and *Involving Patients and the Public in Healthcare*[9] developed this further by giving patients and the public a greater say in the NHS and setting out proposals for implementing patient-centred care. Patient advice and liaison services (PALS) and patient forums were also introduced in every NHS trust. Of particular significance is the Health and Social Care Act 2001; section 11 placed a legal duty on the NHS to involve and consult with patients and the public in planning and delivering health services. This duty was strengthened under section 242 of the National Health Service Act 2006, which also placed a requirement on strategic health authorities, NHS trusts, NHS foundation trusts and primary care trusts to involve patients and the public in planning and developing services.

The emphasis on patient-centred and patient-led services and public engagement remained central to government policy in subsequent moves to modernise services.[7,11,17,18] Foundation trusts and the introduction of local involvement networks further increased public scrutiny of NHS business and the accountability of service providers. However, despite the wealth of policy and guidance, PPI has lacked consistency in its application as confirmed by the *Health Committee's Report on Patient and Public Involvement in the NHS* in 2007.[13] The report stated that the purpose of PPI was not clear in relation to improving the design and provision of services and increasing accountability.

Incorporating policy on engagement into strategy affecting people with dementia using health and social care services has been most evident through the National Dementia Strategy,[2] which has a number of objectives that support increased inclusion of people with dementia and their carers.

➤ *Objective 5* – advocates developing peer support and learning networks in local areas to provide practical and emotional support and promote self-care. This could result in a reduction in social isolation and could also be a source of information for commissioners of services.

➤ *Objective 11* – living well with dementia in care homes outlines the need for care homes to enhance relationships with relatives to reduce carers' stress.

➤ *Objective 14* – states that joint commissioning strategies need to recognise that a person's health and social care needs do not remain static and will change over time. It recommends that outcomes should be developed with service users and their carers.

Engagement is monitored by the Care Quality Commission (formed in April 2009), which inspects the quality of health and social care services. It will assess the progress of the National Dementia Strategy and as part of this will assess the experience of service users through discussion, observations and links with carers.

Similarly, the earlier guidance produced by the National Institute for Health and Clinical Excellence in 2006 advocated including service users and carers in joint planning between health and social care services. The National Service Framework for Older People[19] also supported older people being allowed to make choices about their own care. Personalisation and self-directed care, introduced in 2007 through Putting People First[20] reforms to provision of social care, are intended to empower the service user and increase their control and choice over the services they receive. However, as with any PPE, there is a tendency to focus on the process of engagement rather than outcomes, hence the findings of Law *et al.*[1] that evidence of change in service delivery and at a strategic level is limited.

Moreover, the National Audit Office,[21] whilst acknowledging that there had been significant spending on dementia by both health and social care services, felt that intervention was not early enough. Its view was that early interventions were effective and improved quality of life but were not introduced early enough, increasing spending later when more services were needed and were more expensive. The report recommended involving older people with dementia and their carers locally in developing joint needs analyses and local area agreements.

MODELS AND APPROACHES TO ENGAGEMENT

The stated vision for health and social care providers is:

> ... for patients and the public to drive the design and delivery of high-quality services.

> (Department of Health 2009[22])

In order to achieve this vision, the aspiration was for health and social care professionals to work with service users, carers and the public, to offer service users opportunities for involvement in order to share their experience of services and to use their experience to influence services. By excluding people with dementia from playing a part in developing and improving services, we discriminate and oppress, marginalise and restrict the right to person-centred, self-directed care. However, in working towards engagement we have to recognise a holistic model of the person with social, economic, housing and spiritual needs as well as health needs. Services have to be culturally sensitive and relevant, which means being aware of language issues, beliefs and practices related to culture, identity and support needs. Involving older people with dementia in service planning, development and delivery will increase the awareness of policy makers and health and social care workers and could bridge the gap between policy and practice.

Having the knowledge, expertise and experience of people who are living with dementia and how dementia affects a person's life can enhance the relevance and inclusivity of services and further co-production. The benefits of involving service users and carers in the planning and delivery of health services, including through the education and training of professionals, and research have been well documented.[23–27] Benefits include:

➤ learning from the knowledge and perspective of service users and carers of living with and managing health problems and using services
➤ challenging professional perspectives
➤ valuing of the service user and carer perspective
➤ development of new skills and knowledge for both professionals and service users and carers
➤ development of a greater understanding of health services and professional training for the service user or carer
➤ improving understanding of the carer's role, identifying the most appropriate services and gaps in services, driving up standards and quality.

Other impacts of engagement can be a reduction of the stigma and discrimination experienced by those with dementia. Raising the profile of the lived experience has the potential to reduce the fear factor and myths surrounding the illness. No less important are the personal benefits of engagement for the person with dementia or their carers; this may include increased feelings of empowerment, being valued, improved self-esteem and improved physical and mental well-being.[28] Participation and engagement, including voluntary activity, will increase the potential to live an active life and, if the engagement activity involves meeting others, increases inclusion and reduces social exclusion.[29,30] Peer support can be an important facet of social inclusion.

Barriers to engagement include:

➤ professionals and organisations having the time and resources to devote to meaningful participation
➤ health and social care staff not recognising that people with dementia have the ability to participate
➤ health and social care structures for communicating being largely based on a formula of meetings and electronic means which rarely produce information in accessible formats
➤ service users' fear of being labelled as service users if they agree to involvement; they and their carers may have concerns about speaking out and being seen as critical of services and thereby affecting their care or the treatment of the person being cared for.

Additional barriers exist for hard to reach groups, for example, black and minority ethnic communities and disabled groups, who may not know where to access information about available services.

Achieving meaningful engagement

People with dementia are a diverse group of people and whilst they share some experience they also have individual concerns and needs. These concerns and needs do not simply relate to healthcare as social and other needs are also crucial. Meaningful engagement starts from recognising the important role that older adults play in society, in families and as carers. Engagement may start at an individual (egoist) level with participation in care planning, decisions about treatment, choice and managing direct payments;[31,32] or may be more altruistic and take the form of participation in a support, advocacy or lobbying group or charitable foundation. Research into participation has tended to focus on the extent of engagement (using a model such as Arnstein's 'ladder of participation'[33]); however, the level of engagement is not necessarily the issue if the principle of inclusion is based on responsiveness to needs and empowerment and choice for the service user and carer. To be effective, engagement on any level must have meaning in the person's life and lead to positive outcomes on a personal or more general level. Of equal importance is the impact of involvement on service development. The older people's inquiry into 'That Bit of Help'[34] concluded that unless service users are involved, developments are unlikely to be long lasting. Others have concluded that research, information sheets, books or web resources developed by people with experience are likely to have more resonance with their peers.[35,36]

Participation, power, choice and control are facilitated by the provision of good quality information, consultation, engagement in decision making and support. To increase social inclusion, it is important to recognise the need to work with local communities and integrate opportunities for older adults into provision. Ageing can lead to social isolation and this can be compounded by developing an affective disorder, which might lead to the person withdrawing from social contact. One response to this has been to extend the Sure Start programme for families to older adults through Link-Age Plus,[37,38] which aimed to reduce social exclusion and poverty.

Approaches to engagement

In addition to the different levels of participation outlined by Arnstein (Arnstein's ladder of participation has eight rungs ranging from 1, manipulation through consultation, partnership, to 8, citizen control) and others[39,40] there are, arguably, different levels of service user engagement within each of those, ranging from passive to active participation. With people with dementia, it has often been passive participation. The Social Care Institute for Excellence[37] outlines two approaches to participation: (i) discrete activity; (ii) participation as part of everyday activities, i.e. service delivery. The authors concluded that an integrated approach was the most effective in engaging seldom heard groups such as those with dementia. This approach was achieved through building strong relationships between staff and service users, being inclusive regardless of the motivation for involvement and including people at the centre of the process. The outcomes of this were joint problem solving, improvements to policy and practice and increased confidence for service users and carers.

Specifically in relation to dementia services, Cantley *et al.*[36] identified four categories of approach when involving people with dementia: individual consultation, group consultation, participation and collective action. The authors also identified some principles for engaging with older people with dementia – seeing the person as a whole person with different dimensions, i.e. emotional, spiritual, social, and not focusing on cognitive ability. They advocated valuing the person's citizenship and working towards social inclusion, empowerment and choice.

For those who should be considering engagement, i.e. commissioners of services, health, social care and third sector providers/practitioners, *Understanding What Matters*[42] provides guidance on using feedback based on service user experience to ensure quality improvement. The emphasis on experience, rather than satisfaction, marked a shift from the satisfaction surveys traditionally used as a measure of service evaluation. Although service user and carer engagement has most frequently been initiated by health and social care providers, commissioners can gain a great deal from involving service users and carers. Competency 3 of *World Class Commissioning* directed commissioners to:

> Proactively seek and build continuous and meaningful engagement with the public and patients, to shape services and improve outcomes.[43]

Health and social care commissioners working together with service users and carers to meet needs can do a great deal to ensure joined-up services.

As already indicated, there is a range of ways to involve and engage people; at an individual level involvement in decisions about the person's own care package, self-directed care or personal budgets. There may be opportunities to engage in consultations, for example, NICE guidance,[44] take part in national programmes such as the Alzheimer's Society initiative 'Living with Dementia'. More locally, consultation with individual service users or carers or groups about policy, strategy or service changes may take place.[34] Membership of formal policy or strategy committees enables the service user and/or carer voice to be directly incorporated into developments. Even more formal examples of involvement are when service users or carers are employed as engagement, advocacy or support workers. This type of role might include awareness-raising campaigns, lobbying for change or recruiting community champions. Access to the service user and carer experience might be through the use of focus groups, one-off events, through existing groups or via the internet.[22,45,1] Other forms of engagement might include involvement in research and evaluation (see the Dementias and Neurodegenerative Diseases Research Network, DeNDRoN,[4] a National Institute for Health Research clinical research network facilitating and supporting research in those areas, and Alzheimer's Research Trust), recruitment of staff or education of health and social care staff. Older adults, and older adults' champions, involved in the training of practitioners and clinicians can have the additional benefit of providing positive role models that disprove ageist myths about older adults being passive recipients of services. Similarly, young people's groups such as the People Relying on People Group (PROP) can act as change agents and awareness raisers.[48]

With any form of public engagement, there is a need for staff development to enable this process to happen, but this is even more important with groups with specific issues such as people with dementia. Apart from training and awareness raising, organisations could give consideration to having champions within a staff group. It is also crucial to recognise the ethical issues present when working with vulnerable groups and to ensure consent, for any engagement activity, is in place. Power relationships may be more of a concern where there are issues of capacity as with people with advanced dementia. Power is a complex concept, but it is clearly something that may be a barrier to engagement, particularly in dementia care where the relationship current service users, and carers, have with a clinician, or other health or social care professional, may be affected by the sometimes coercive nature of treatment or dependency on care.

WHAT DO PEOPLE WITH DEMENTIA WANT?

People with dementia are a diverse group and as such will have a diverse range of wishes, but all will require holistic, joined-up services meeting their health and social care needs and reflecting the need to retain their social inclusion. Younger people with dementia are more likely to be economically active and have financial and, potentially, family commitments at the time of onset. Involvement activity may seem more of an anathema to this group unlike the older population who have had time to engage and have more experience of health and social care services. However, quality of life may not be seen as predominant for the older population, who are viewed as needing care rather than being encouraged in techniques for self-care. The Joseph Rowntree Foundation[31] suggests that policy and practice in services for older adults is framed in the context of two models: deficit and heroic. The deficit model sees old age as an incurable illness where older adults are the passive recipients of care. Decisions about care and treatment are taken by professionals and, when ill, older adults experience a loss of control and power. The heroic model cites successful ageing as the ability to remain on a physical par with younger people. Neither of these models represents the reality for the majority of older adults who wish to play an active role in the community and retain a reasonable quality of life.

Information is crucial to any engagement activity, whether it be individual or collective, to enable choice and engagement. Older people, in particular, want to remain independent and would like help to do so and to remain at home and in the community. Creative solutions are sometimes needed to allow people to retain their independence and also take part in service development. As the use of telemedicine/telecare becomes more prevalent this can be a means of communication as well as a potential way to avoid long-term residential care. People with dementia want to make their own decisions wherever possible.

In common with most consumers, older adults want choice when accessing the services they require. This ideal underpins much of recent public sector reform, particularly in the NHS.[49,11,22,17,18] The evidence is that increased choice of care and treatment and involvement in care planning increases satisfaction with services and encourages self-management, but this is a complex area as it depends on the availability of a range of services, the ability and capacity to make relevant choices and the willingness of clinicians and professionals to accept the choices of service users and carers.[50,51] Organisational culture may also need to shift to facilitate a greater level of engagement or co-production in the planning and delivery of services,[52,53] but is predicated on the understanding of the service user and/or carer's motives for involvement. Moreover, service user engagement in mental health services is patchy, with an emphasis on consultation rather than influence, partnership or control. Care homes are often regarded as unlikely environments for engaging with people, but Cantley and Wilson[54] suggest that the best homes had managers who were open to involving residents and families in the management of the homes.

Older adults and their carers want holistic and flexible services that respond to their practical, physical and psychological needs. They also want culturally relevant services that are based in the community and reflect local needs. The voluntary sector can play a key role in the provision of services, especially day services, and engage with people with dementia, particularly if they can work within local communities. Community groups, such as faith-based groups, could also play a key role in engaging members of the community and reducing social isolation. Older adults will welcome safe environments where they can receive psychological and emotional support and some will appreciate provision for their spiritual needs. Local services increase social inclusion as those older adults with mobility issues, whether through physical or mental ill health, are unlikely to travel outside their community to access services.

GOOD PRACTICE GUIDANCE FOR ENGAGING PEOPLE WITH DEMENTIA

Engaging with people with dementia, particularly those who may be past the early stages of the disease, will require careful planning in order to empower the service user and carer and allow them to communicate their views and needs. Treating them with dignity and respect and safeguarding their rights and interests is fundamental. It is imperative that health and social care staff operate at a pace that the service user or carer wants to work at, this may need to be slower than usual to allow time to think about or formulate a response. Creative methods of engagement and different tools may be needed as processing lots of information might be difficult, for example, use of arts or visual techniques, etc. Big or long meetings may be difficult if there is a lot of information to process or a lot of discussion, and concentration may only last for a short time. Relationship building and communication is central to the success of engagement and, when working with service users with dementia, listening, observing and giving prompts where needed are important. Feedback is important to communicate the value of involvement to the individual and how it will be incorporated into service development.

Consideration should be given to the environment in which engagement activity takes place as this may need to be calm and without distractions. Information is necessary to enable the person to take part and to influence and shape services. The support and resources needed to allow the service user or carer to engage should be considered. This may be practical support, such as transport, expenses, providing notes in easy-to-read formats, arranging for someone to meet the person or allowing them to bring someone with them to a meeting, or may involve mentoring and training. In rural areas transport may be an issue if there are less amenities and public services. A Cabinet Office report in 2009[55] estimated that the rate of dementia will grow faster in rural than urban areas over next decade, with social care needs also projected to grow faster, so hearing the voice of those people is important.

It is possible that a person's condition may deteriorate and they can no longer participate in the way they have done in the past. In these circumstances it may be possible to work towards a solution and enable participation in another way if the person wishes.

CONCLUSIONS

Although the role of service users and carers in the management of dementia is still developing, it is clear that there are already areas where engagement leads to real achievements. The achievements can be identified as those pertinent to the individual service user and carer, i.e. improved well-being, increased self-esteem and feeling valued. Service users and carers also contribute to the knowledge base, which in turn leads to the development of more relevant services. This has been important in the development of good practice and the recognition of the most effective methods of involving people with dementia. However, involving people with dementia in future health and social care service development has inherent challenges in an era of finite resources, service reform, efficiency savings and the drive for better quality services. Policy direction and the wishes of people with dementia may not necessarily be co-terminous. Service users and carers may, for example, want to focus on early intervention but limited resources mean treatment is limited to those with the highest dependency. Commissioning arrangements and privatisation of some care provision may also dilute the potential influence of service users and carers. Despite the resource implications of achieving meaningful engagement with service users and carers, it is more critically important then ever, in an era of public service cuts, that they have a voice and influence service development to ensure resources are used effectively and lead to improved outcomes for the service user.

Key points

➤ UK health and social care policy clearly indicates that service users and carers should be involved in the planning and delivery of services.

➤ Personalisation and self-directed care are intended to empower the service user and increase their control and choice over the services they receive.

➤ Service users and carers can share their experience of care and treatment and play a part in developing and improving services.

➤ To ensure the meaningful engagement of people with dementia, a range of methods and techniques may be employed to facilitate communication.

➤ Staff training is crucial to successful engagement.

➤ There can be real benefits to engagement for service development, including improved understanding and knowledge of the service user experience, and a challenge to professional perspectives.

➤ There can be real benefits to engagement for the service user and carer, including improved self-esteem and confidence, physical and mental well-being and a reduction in social exclusion.

REFERENCES

1 Law S, Janzon K. Engaging older people in reviewing the influence of service users on the quality and delivery of social care services. *Research Policy and Planning*. 2004; 22: 2.

2   Department of Health. *Living Well with Dementia: a national dementia strategy.* London: DoH; 2009.

3   Age Concern England. *Improving services and support for older people with mental health problems. The second report from the UK Inquiry into Mental Health and Well-being in Later Life.* Age Concern England; 2007.

4   Anderson D, Banerjee S, Barker A, *et al. The Need to Tackle Age Discrimination in Mental Health. A compendium of evidence.* London: Royal College of Psychiatrists; 2009.

5   Department of Health. *In the Public Interest: developing a strategy for public participation in the NHS.* London: DoH; 1998.

6   Department of Health. *Patient and Public Involvement in the New NHS.* London: DoH; 1999.

7   Department of Health. *NHS Plan.* London: DoH; 2000.

8   Health and Social Care Act 2001. Available at: www.legislation.gov.uk/ukpga/2001/15/contents (accessed May 2011).

9   Department of Health. *Involving Patients and the Public in Health Care.* London: DoH; 2001.

10 Department of Health. *NHS Improvement Plan.* London: DoH; 2004.

11 Department of Health. *Creating a Patient Led NHS.* London: DoH; 2005.

12 Department of Health. *Reward and Recognition.* London: DoH; 2006.

13 Department of Health. *Health Committee's Report on Patient and Public Involvement in the NHS.* London: DoH; 2007.

14 Bowers H, Eastman M, Harris J, *et al. Moving Out of the Shadows. A report on mental health and wellbeing in later life.* Bournemouth: Help and Care Development Ltd; 2005.

15 Petch, A. *Intermediate Care: what do we know about older people's experiences?* York: Joseph Rowntree Foundation; 2003.

16 Quinn A, Snowling A, Denicolo P. *Older People's Perspectives: devising information, advice and advocacy services.* York: Joseph Rowntree Foundation; 2003.

17 Department of Health. *Equity and Excellence: liberating the NHS.* Norwich: The Stationery Office Ltd; 2010.

18 Department of Health. *A Vision for Adult Social Care: capable communities and active citizens.* The Stationery Office Ltd; 2010.

19 Department of Health. *National Service Framework for Older People.* London: DoH; 2001.

20 Department of Health. *Putting People First: a shared vision and commitment to the transformation of adult social care.* London: DoH; 2007.

21 National Audit Office. *Improving Services and Support for People with Dementia.* London: The Stationery Office; 2007.

22 Department of Health. *Putting Patients at the Heart of Care. The vision for patient and public engagement in health and social care.* London: DoH; 2009.

23 Happell B, Roper C. The role of a mental health consumer in the education of postgraduate psychiatric nursing students: the student's evaluation. *Journal of Psychiatric and Mental Health Nursing.* 2003; **10**, 343–50.

24 Bennett L, Baikie K. The client as educator: learning about mental illness through the eyes of the expert. *Nurse Education Today.* 2003; **23**(2): 104–11.

25 Khoo R, McVicar A, Brandon D. Service user involvement in postgraduate mental

health education. Does it benefit practice? *Journal of Mental Health*. 2004; **13**(5): 481–92.

26 Staley K, Minogue V. User involvement leads to more ethically sound research. *Clinical Ethics*. 2006; **1**: 95–100.

27 Wallcraft J, Schrank B, Amering M. *Handbook of Service User Involvement in Mental Health Research*. Chichester: Wiley-Blackwell; 2009.

28 Lorentzon M, Bryan K. Respect for the person with dementia: fostering greater user involvement in service planning. *Quality in Ageing*. 2007; **8**(1): 23–30.

29 Godfrey M, Townsend J, Surr C, *et al. Prevention and Service Provision: mental health problems in later life*. Institute of Health Services and Public Health Research, Leeds University and Division of Dementia Studies, Bradford University; 2005.

30 Allen J. *Older People and Wellbeing*. London: Institute for Public Policy Research; 2008.

31 Joseph Rowntree Foundation. *Older People Shaping Policy and Practice*. York: Joseph Rowntree Foundation; 2004.

32 Heslop P. *Direct Payment for Mental Health Users/Survivors. A guide to some key issues*. London: National Centre for Independent Living; 2005.

33 Arnstein SR. A ladder of citizen participation. *Journal of the American Planning Association*. 1969; **35**(4): 216–24.

34 Raynes N, Clark H, Beecham J. *The Report of the Older People's Inquiry into 'That Bit of Help'*. York: Joseph Rowntree Foundation; 2006.

35 Crawford M, Rutter D, Thelwall S. *User Involvement in Change Management: a review of the literature*. Report to the National Co-ordinating Centre for NHS Service Delivery and Organisation (NCCSDO); 2003.

36 Cantley C, Woodhouse J, Smith M. *Listen to Us: involving people with dementia in planning and developing services*. Newcastle: Dementia North, Northumbria University; 2005

37 Department for Communities and Local Government. 2006. www.communities. gov.uk/index.asp?id (accessed May 2011).

38 Davis H, Ritters K. *LinkAge Plus National Evaluation: end of project report*. Department for Work and Pensions Research Report No 572. Norwich: The Stationery Office; 2009.

39 Collins K, Ison R. *Dare We Jump Off Arnstein's Ladder? Social learning as a new policy paradigm.* Buckingham: Open University Press; 2006.

40 Tritter JQ, McCallum A. The snakes and ladders of user involvement: moving beyond Arnstein. *Health Policy*. 2006; **76**: 156–68.

41 Social Care Institute for Excellence. *Seldom Heard: developing inclusive participation in social care*. London: SCIE; 2008.

42 Department of Health. *Understanding What Matters*. London: DoH; 2009.

43 Department of Health. *World Class Commissioning Competencies*. London: DoH; 2007.

44 National Institute for Health and Clinical Excellence. *Dementia. Supporting people with dementia and their carers in health and social care: NICE guideline 42*. London: NIHCE; 2006. www.nice.org.uk/guidance/CG042

45 Astell A, Alm N, Gowans G, *et al.* Involving older people with dementia and their carers in designing computer based support systems: some methodological considerations. *Univ Access Inf Soc*. 2009; **8**: 49–58.

46 Dementias and Neurodegenerative Diseases Research Network (DeNDRoN), www. dendron.org.uk (accessed May 2011).

47 Alzheimer's Research Trust, http://curealzfund.org/research (accessed May 2011).

48 Department of Health and National Institute for Mental Health in England. *User and Carer Involvement in Dementia Care.* London: DoH; 2005.

49 Department of Health. *High Quality Care for All: NHS next stage review final report.* London: DoH; 2008.

50 Department of Health. *Patient and Public Involvement in Health: the evidence for policy implementation. A summary of the results of the Health in Partnership research programme.* London: HMSO; 2004.

51 Department of Health. *Better Information, Better Choices, Better Health: putting information at the centre of health.* London: HMSO; 2004.

52 Hyde P, Davies, HTO. Service design, culture and performance in health services: consumers as co-producers. *Human Relations.* 2004; **11**: 1407–26.

53 Boyle D, Burns S, Conisbee M. *Towards and Asset-based NHS.* London: New Economics Foundation; 2004.

54 Cantley C, Wilson R. *Designing and Managing Care Homes for People with Dementia.* York: Joseph Rowntree Foundation; 2002.

55 Cabinet Office Social Exclusion Task Force. *Working Together for Older People in Rural Areas.* London: Cabinet Office; 2009.

Index